Y0-CAO-080

Fifteenth in the SPIE Critical Reviews of Technology Series

Volume 604

Holographic Nondestructive Testing: Status and Comparison with Conventional Methods

Charles M. Vest
Chairman/Editor

Presented in cooperation with
American Association of Physicists in Medicine • Center for Applied Optics/University of Alabama in Huntsville
Center for Laser Studies/University of Southern California • Georgia Institute of Technology
Institute of Optics/University of Rochester • Laser Association of America
Office of Naval Research • Optical Sciences Center/University of Arizona

23–24 January 1986
Los Angeles, California

An SPIE Critical Reviews of Technology conference brings together an invited group of experts in a selected technology. Each presents an extended critical review paper that characterizes the state of the art of the technology by assessing key developments from past research and identifying important areas of current work. The conference is designed to present an overview of the technology and to result in a proceedings of value to individuals working in this or related technologies.

Published by
SPIE—The International Society for Optical Engineering
P.O. Box 10, Bellingham, Washington 98227-0010 USA
Telephone 206/676-3290 (Pacific Time) • Telex 46-7053

SPIE (The Society of Photo-Optical Instrumentation Engineers) is a nonprofit society dedicated to advancing engineering and scientific applications of optical, electro-optical, and optoelectronic instrumentation, systems, and technology.

The papers appearing in this book comprise the proceedings of the meeting mentioned on the cover and title page. They reflect the authors' opinions and are published as presented and without change, in the interests of timely dissemination. Their inclusion in this publication does not necessarily constitute endorsement by the editors or by SPIE.

Please use the following format to cite material from this book:
Author(s), "Title of Paper," *Holographic Nondestructive Testing: Status and Comparison with Conventional Methods,* Charles M. Vest, Editor, Proc. SPIE 604, page numbers (1986).

Library of Congress Catalog Card No. 86-070342
ISBN 0-89252-639-4

Printed in the United States of America.

HOLOGRAPHIC NONDESTRUCTIVE TESTING:
STATUS AND COMPARISON WITH CONVENTIONAL METHODS

Volume 604

Contents

HOLOGRAPHIC NONDESTRUCTIVE TESTING:
STATUS AND COMPARISON WITH CONVENTIONAL METHODS

Volume 604

INTRODUCTION

This critical review of holographic nondestructive testing was held in Los Angeles in January 1986. The goal was to assess the technical status of holographic NDT and to provide comparative technical and economic evaluation of holographic and nonholographic NDT methods. Review papers were presented by an international panel of experts having a wide variety of relevant backgrounds, including involvement in state-of-the-art research on holographic interferometry and related optical techniques, experience with conventional NDT methods, and involvement with competing developing technologies.

The session was opened by George Birnbaum who provided a rather broad perspective by surveying a range of optical NDE activities at the U.S. National Bureau of Standards. This opening paper provided a context within which the review papers dealing with specific holographic and speckle techniques and applications were set. Conclusions regarding these techniques varied greatly according to application area. A particularly interesting objective analysis of holographic and nonholographic techniques for testing associated with nuclear power plants was presented by David Mader, who concluded that for his particular applications other techniques were more appropriate. On the other hand, John Newman and others presented some very successful routine industrial applications of holographic NDT. Unique features of holographic interferometry for quantitative analysis of very small mechanical and electronic components were illustrated by Ryszard Pryputniewicz. John Tyrer and Y. Y. Hung illustrated interesting applications of the related technologies of electronic speckle pattern interferometry and shearography.

A number of areas in which improvements of the technology would be valuable were pointed out, but in general there was considerable indication that while holographic NDT is unlikely to become a generally applicable "black box" NDT technique, there do exist a number of particular problem areas for which it is uniquely qualified. Modest but increasing industrial application should be anticipated, particularly as our ability to quantitatively and automatically interpret results increases.

Charles M. Vest
University of Michigan

Optical nondestructive evaluation at the National Bureau of Standards

G. Birnbaum*, D. Nyyssonen**, C. M. Vest***, and T. V. Vorburger*

*National Bureau of Standards, Gaithersburg, Maryland 20899, respectively,
Office of Nondestructive Evaluation and Mechanical Production Metrology Division
**CD Metrology, Inc., Germantown, MD 20874
***College of Engineering, The University of Michigan, Ann Arbor, Michigan 48109-2092

Abstract

This report reviews recent and current work on a variety of optical techniques applied to nondestructive evaluation (NDE) and carried out by the National Bureau of Standards. The optical methods discussed include holography, scattering from surfaces, microscopy, scattering from particles, and methods employing optical fibers. Much of this work is aimed at the development of accurate measurement methods for in-service inspection and for process monitoring in manufacturing, and at the development of standards and calibration procedures.

1. Introduction

This review deals with a variety of optical techniques applied to nondestructive evaluation (NDE) and carried out at, or supported by, the National Bureau of Standards (NBS). The research programs described here were developed independently in various divisions of NBS as responses to NDE problems deemed to be solvable by optical technology. What makes some aspects of this work unique to NBS is the emphasis given to the development of accurate measurement methods, standards, and calibration procedures.

The optical NDE methods discussed here include holography (Section 2), scattering from surfaces (Section 3), microscopy (Section 4), scattering from particles (Section 5), and methods employing optical fibers (Section 6). All these techniques employ a laser source and, with a single exception, the scattered or imaged laser radiation was analyzed to obtain the information relevant to NDE. This employment of lasers in NDE should be contrasted with that where the laser is used as a transducer to generate ultrasonic and thermal waves which probe the sample and are analyzed for NDE-related information [1,2]. Section 2 describes some exploratory work aimed at increasing the ease of flaw dectection by holography and at measuring simultaneously surface displacement and tilt in real time. Section 3 discusses the measurement of scattering from metallic surfaces to characterize quantitatively surface roughness. Section 4 discusses a relatively mature program, the use of optical microscopy for the accurate measurement of the width of lines on photomasks and wafers. Section 5 deals with the determination of liquid droplet size, velocity, and concentration. Section 6 presents some novel uses of optical fibers in NDE applications. These sections contain a description of the techniques and their applications to NDE problems. Some plans for future work are mentioned.

2. Holographic methods

Digital and optical moiré detection of flaws

The objective of this work is to increase the ease of flaw detection by holographic nondestructive testing (HNDT). Most commonly, holographic NDT tests are made by a double exposure method. During the first exposure of the hologram the test object is in an initial undeformed state, and during the second exposure it is subjected to some appropriate state of stress. The output of such a double exposure process is an interferogram, i.e., an image of the object modulated by a set of interference fringes indicative of the deformation of the object between exposures. Under appropriate conditions, the presence of a flaw in the object is manifested as a change in this fringe pattern relative to that of a nominally identical object without a flaw. If the flaw only leads to a small perturbation of this fringe pattern, it may be difficult to detect, particularly by an unskilled operator.

If a transparency of the interference pattern of a flawed object is superimposed on the interference pattern from a nominally identical object without a flaw, a broad moiré pattern will be seen. This moiré pattern is indicative of differences between the two interferograms. Although simple in principle, this method of flaw detection is difficult in practice because the clamping and stressing of the test object and the flaw-free object must be virtually identical so that object deformations are essentially the same to within a few wavelengths of light. This condition may be met in the laboratory, but it is unlikely to be achieved in industrial applications. If this is not the case, confusing extraneous moiré patterns may confuse the operator. In an attempt to alleviate this problem, three techniques are used for improving moiré detection of flaws: (1) introducing a small relative magnification of the transparencies of the flawed and flaw-free objects in order to compensate for small differences in stress level; (2) forming a moiré pattern by superimposing two transparencies of a single interferogram of the flawed component, which differ only by a small relative magnification; and (3) utilizing digital imaging processing to form and enhance the moiré patterns of techniques (1) and (2).

In order to explore these techniques both analytically and experimentally, it was desirable to work with a test object yielding a rather simple fringe pattern. The particular test objects in these experiments were flat aluminum disks of 15 cm diameter and 6.3 mm thickness. The "flaws" were flat-bottomed slots of various depths, aspect ratios, locations, and orientations, machined into the back surfaces of the disks. Each disk was clamped around its periphery, and nitrogen gas was used to apply a uniform pressure over its back surface. Two-exposure holographic interferograms were recorded with a pressure change of typically 40 kPa between the exposures. This configuration leads to a set of fringes which ideally are perfectly circular and concentric in the case of a flaw-free object.

A moiré pattern was formed by superimposing one interferogram of such an object with two flaws and one of a flaw-free object subjected to slightly different pressure. Although moiré fringes were seen indicating the presence of the two flaws, the pattern was cluttered by extraneous, approximately circular, moiré fringes. These are due to the fact that the pressure difference was slightly different in the two cases. Figure 1 was formed in the same manner as described above; however, a slight relative magnification of the transparencies was used to compensate for the slight pressure difference. There are two oval-shaped flaws--one above the center which is oriented horizontally, and one below the center

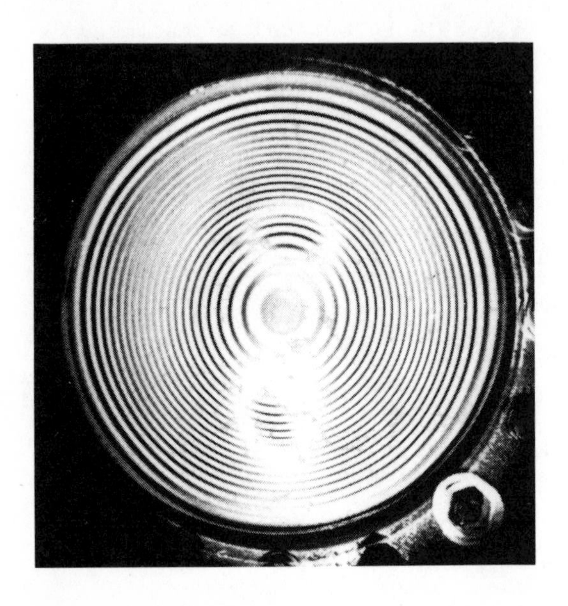

Figure 1. Optical superposition of two similar interferograms, one with a slight relative magnification to correct for unequal pressure (loading) differences. The interferogram is that of an aluminum disk with two flaws and a similar disk which is flaw free, subjected to a slightly different pressure. Closed moiré fringes outline the flaws (from Reference 3).

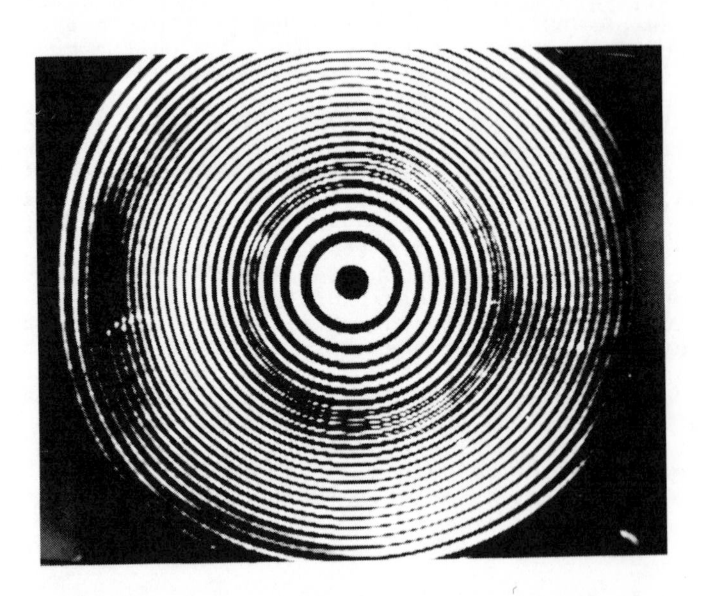

Figure 2. Computer superposition of the same interferogram but with a relative magnification of 1.04. A single, two-exposure interferogram of a flawed disk was digitized and a second image, identical with the first but magnified, was computed. Their product was formed and displayed. The flaw appears as a black moiré fringe at the left (from Reference 3).

which is inclined somewhat to the vertical. The region of high contrast fringes inside each of the moiré fringes define the size and shape of the flaws. At least in the case of a simple symmetrical pattern, this technique can produce an excellent indication of sufficiently large flaws and give a reasonable indication of their size and shape. However, it is quite cumbersome in practice and may require trial and error to determine the appropriate magnification, although some analysis has been done to estimate it [3].

In order to improve the usefulness of this technique, methods were explored which required the use of only a single interferogram, i.e., that of a differentially pressured, flawed test object. In these experiments the flaws led to rather subtle perturbations of the basic concentric circular fringe pattern and were difficult to detect by the unaided eye. In particular, flaws tangent to the basic fringe pattern were extremely difficult to see. However, a moiré pattern formed by superimposing an interferogram of a flawed test object and a transparency of the same fringe pattern, magnified by a few percent, clearly indicated the flaw.

Although the approach of forming a moiré pattern from two identical interferograms, with one being slightly magnified relative to the other, will work, there are several problems with it. In particular, the technique depends upon having simple symmetrical basic fringe patterns. Also, the exact magnification required to produce a clear indication of the flaw may vary from region to region of the interferogram. Finally, the process of producing and superimposing the two interferograms is quite cumbersome. In order to alleviate these difficulties, the formation of moiré fringes by digital computation was explored. The single, two-exposure interferogram of the flawed test object was digitized by a 512 x 512 pixel solid-state array camera and was stored in a computer memory. A second image, identical with the first but magnified by a factor of 1.04, was computed and stored. A bias level was introduced by subtracting the same constant from each image to avoid saturation; the images were then multiplied and their product displayed on a video monitor as shown in Figure 2. The flaw appears as a black moiré fringe at the left of the disk.

This work has indicated that at least in fairly ideal circumstances, moiré patterns can be formed in various ways from holographic interferograms and used to display flaws. The most significant part of this work is the concept of using digital image processing to form the moiré pattern from a single interferogram. This technique has significant potential and should be explored further. In particular, the power of digital image analysis allows one to apply a variety of transformations to the interferogram in addition to the simple magnification used here. One can envision a system whereby the operator could rapidly explore a variety of magnifications, stretchings, or other transformations, and examine an interferogram region by region until a clear indication of the presence or absence of flaws is seen. A wide variety of such operations could be carried out and many filtering, enhancement, and display techniques also could be used.

Point holography for simultaneous measurement of displacement and tilt

A technique has been developed whereby holographic interferometry can be used to simultaneously measure dynamically, i.e., in real time, displacement, tilt, and in some circumstances in-plane displacement of the region near a point on an object surface. Generally, holographic interferometry is used to produce whole-field visualizations or measurements of surface displacements. Analysis of whole-field interferograms to determine quantities such as displacement or tilt involves use of the entire image and sometimes relatively complicated computation. Here holographic interferometry is used in a very different way in order to monitor the motion of a small region of the surface.

The basic system is shown schematically in Figure 3. Two closely spaced points, P and Q, on the object's surface are illuminated by parallel, unexpanded, or even focused, laser beams at an angle α to the surface normal. Light scattered by the material in the neighborhood of points P and Q at an angle α to the other side of the normal is directed by lenses L_1 and L_2 toward a photodetector D. A holographic recording medium H is placed at some convenient point in this optical system. In the experiments reported here, the recording medium was a photoconductor-thermoplastic plate, 30 mm square.

In this technique, an initial holographic exposure is made while the surface is illuminated by the dual beams and while the object is in some initial static condition. The holographic recording plate is developed and reilluminated both by a reconstruction wave and by light scattered by the dual beams impinging at points P and Q. Thus the detector simultaneously receives the holographically reconstructed light scattered from the points in the initial static condition and the light scattered by the same points as the object is deformed. The lenses and detector should be arranged in such a manner that the detector does not separately resolve the two closely spaced points P and Q. As the experiment proceeds, the electrical output of the photodetector is used to drive some display device, which is a rapidly responsive plotter in this case.

In these experiments, the object was a thick aluminum disk which was being pressurized by nitrogen gas from behind. Figure 4 shows the output signal of the detector as the disk was deformed. The output signal consists of a relatively high-frequency oscillation which is modulated by a more slowly varying envelope structure, and, finally, the entire signal is modulated by an approximately exponential decay.

Analysis [4] shows that the fine structure of this signal indicates the normal displacement of the object's surface with the usual interferometric accuracy. Thus, the high frequency oscillation in Figure 4 can be used to determine normal deformation just as in the case of normal real-time holographic interferometry, Michelson interferometry, or

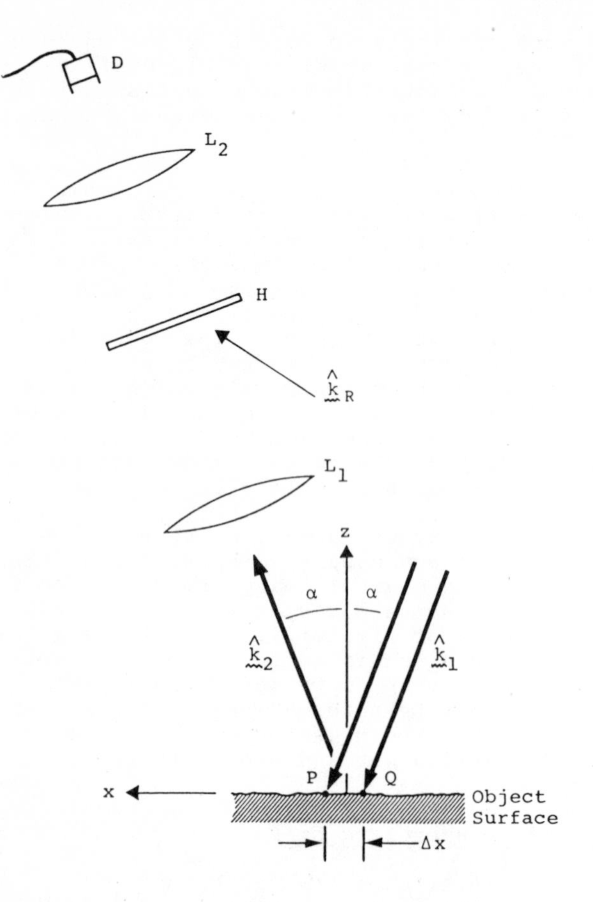

Figure 3. Holographic optical system for simultaneous measurement of displacement and tilt. P and Q are separately illuminated points on the object surface. The imaging system is composed of lenses L_1 and L_2. The hologram is recorded in plane H with a reference wave $\hat{k}_R$, and the points P and Q are imaged onto detector D (from Reference 4).

other similar techniques. The period of the more slowly varying oscillatory envelope is a measure of the amount of tilt, i.e., rotation about a line parallel to the surface, of the object in the vicinity of points P and Q. Finally, the overall decay of the signal is due to decreasing correlation of the light scattered as deformation increases. This decorrelation is indicative of in-plane translation. In this experiment, the spacing between points P and Q was 2.0 mm, and the angle α was 10°. A shift of one fringe in the fine structure corresponds to a normal displacement of 0.32 μm, and each pair of zero crossings of the oscillatory modulation corresponds to a tilt of 0.16 mrad. In general, the in-plane displacement is much less straightforward to determine because it depends on optical decorrelation and therefore somewhat on the microstructure of the material, the wavelength of light, the amount of strain, etc. In principle, an empirical study for a given material and optical configuration might enable one to determine this displacement. It is likely that one can determine whether or not the direction of object motion changes during the experiment. If the motion were to reverse and move back toward the initial state, the magnitude of the oscillations after having decreased, as is the case in Figure 4, would increase.

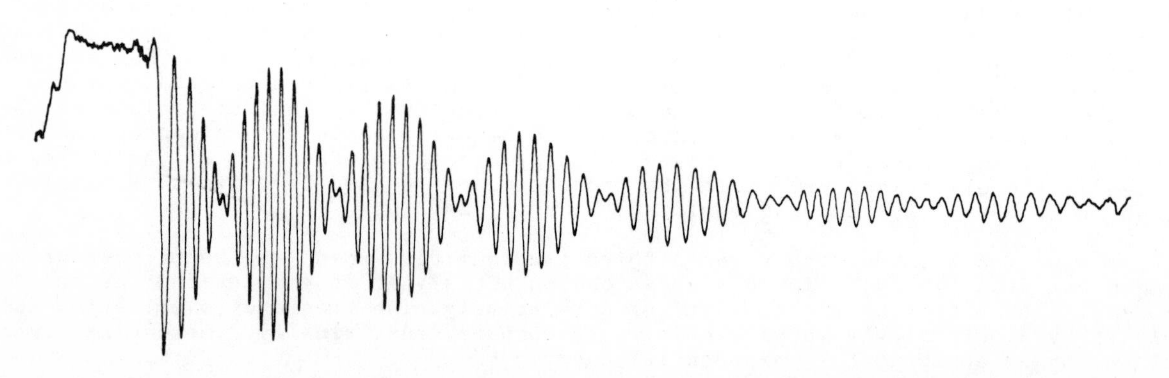

Figure 4. Typical plot of the output signal for Δx = 2.0 mm and for $\alpha = 10^\circ$ (see Figure 3). A shift of one fringe corresponds to a normal displacement of 0.32 μm. Each pair of zero crossings of the modulation corresponds to a tilt of 01.16 mrad (from Reference 4).

This work has indicated that dual-point illumination, real-time holographic interferometry can be used to determine simultaneously the local normal translation and tilt of an object's surface as a function of time. In special cases, one might also be able to determine in-plane displacement. After further development, this technique may be useful for monitoring motions due to transient phenomena such as stress wave propagation. A variety of generalizations of this technique is possible, but that reported here appears to be the most useful.

3. Scattering from surfaces

The research on optical scattering from surfaces discussed here is directed toward the measurement of surface roughness and the characterization of surface flaws. Roughness and flaws are complementary aspects of surface topography. The roughness consists of the numerous peaks and valleys left on the surface by the manufacturing process. The flaws are the occasional and unwanted interruptions of the surface topography [5] caused by problems such as defects in the materials that are uncovered by the manufacturing process.

In the work on roughness, the main interest is the characterization of moderately rough engineering surfaces that might be produced by a machining process such as grinding or diamond turning. The research on defects is primarily directed toward the characterization of scratches on optical quality surfaces. The quantification of scratch standards is an area of importance to the optical industry. Each of these areas is discussed.

Optical measurements of surface roughness

There is a great interest in the metal working and other manufacturing industries for optical techniques to measure surface roughness [6]. The most widespread technique, the stylus, is accurate but slow, partly because it develops surface roughness information through point-by-point measurement of surface height with a high-resolution probe. Since the stylus contacts the surface, there is always the potential for surface damage. By contrast, an area technique like optical scattering probes a macroscopic area of the surface and, moreover, is a noncontacting method. Such optical measurements can potentially yield statistical parameters which are related to surface peaks and valleys. Hence, optical scattering techniques hold great potential for high-speed, on-line measurement of surface roughness that is noncontacting and nondestructive. However, a theoretical model is required in order to deduce roughness parameters from optical scattering quantities.

The general phenomena are well understood. When a beam of light illuminates a surface, the radiation is scattered into an angular distribution [7] according to the laws of physical optics. For very smooth surfaces, most of the light is reflected in the specular direction. As the roughness increases, the intensity of the specular beam decreases and the intensity of the diffuse pattern increases. Therefore, the angular distribution may be used as a descriptor of the surface roughness. The theoretical problems regarding the quantitative measurement of roughness by optical scattering involves questions concerning how to deal with roughness heights that are the same order of magnitude as the wavelength of the light, and what statistical model of the surface roughness can allow the deduction of quantities that characterize geometrical roughness.

This work has concentrated thus far on testing optical scattering theory for moderately rough surfaces with a dominant lay pattern. Such patterns are much rougher in one direction than they are in the perpendicular direction and are obtained, for example, by grinding and hand lapping. The optical model is based on a scalar theory (see references in [8]) that is sometimes termed the phase screen approximation. Figure 5 illustrates the idea. An incident plan wave illuminates a surface, and the only changes in the scattered wave that are considered are those due to the changes in phase because the individual light rays must travel different distances as they are reflected by surface irregularities. This theory is valid for surfaces with moderate slopes and requires that the surface wavelengths be significantly greater than the roughness heights. This theory has been tested by measuring the angular intensity distribution of light scattered from various surfaces of known topography. The results obtained from tests of this approach have been generally quite encouraging.

The angular intensity distribution is measured with an instrument called DALLAS [8] (detector array for laser light angular scattering) that consists of an array of 87 detectors in a semicircular yoke. The detector array can be rotated by using a stepping motor in order to collect nearly the entire hemisphere of scattered radiation, but initial studies have been concerned with light scattered nearly into the plane of incidence by surfaces with a strong lay pattern. This one-dimensional situation simplifies considerably the data collection and the theoretical analysis but still provides a useful test of many of the basic assumptions in the theory. The detailed surface topography is measured by a high resolution diamond stylus instrument interfaced to a minicomputer [8]. The outputs from this system are high-resolution surface profiles represented by 4000 digitized points.

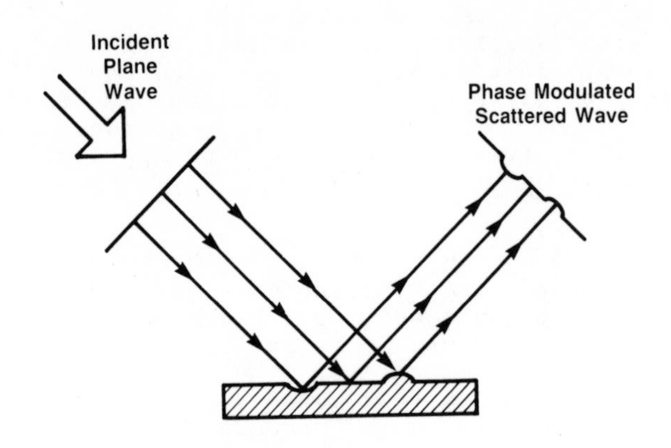

Figure 5. Illustration of the scattering model. The only changes in the scattered wave that are considered are changes in phase because individual light rays travel different distances as they are reflected by surface irregularities.

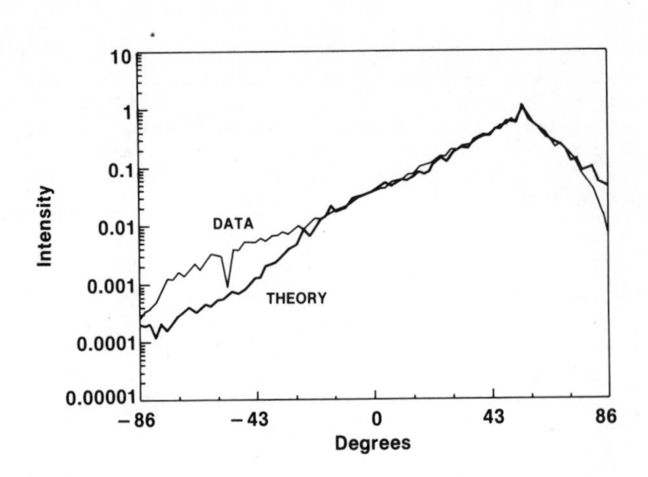

Figure 6. Data obtained from DALLAS [8] compared with a calculation of the scattering from a hand-lapped stainless steel surface with rms roughness equal to 0.22 μm. The angle of incidence of light is -54°.

The first of two experiments, which have been reported previously [8], involved surfaces obtained by grinding. More recently, measurements have been completed on a set of hand-lapped stainless steel specimens with rms roughness ranging from about 0.05 to 0.3 μm. The goal of these measurements was to verify the direct scattering calculations, given the surface topography measured with the stylus instrument. Although the analysis of these results is still in the preliminary stages, the agreement achieved between theory and experiment is quite good, as shown in Figure 6 for a handlapped surface with rms roughness equal to 0.22 μm. Since the angle of incidence is -54°, the angle of specular scattering is +54°, as evidenced by the clear peak in the scattering distribution there. Only in the far left wing of the distribution does the theoretical curve depart significantly from the experimental one. This is likely due to the fact that the stylus instrument has a lateral resolution of only about 0.3 μm. Hence, the high-angle scattering due to such short spatial wavelengths on the surface would not be predicted. Although more work needs to be done, it appears that a straightforward scalar optical theory describes quite well the optical scattering from moderately rough metal surfaces.

Simply accounting for the scattering is not enough; one must also be able to estimate surface roughness characteristics from the scattering data. To accomplish this, it is necessary to use inverse scattering algorithms with appropriate surface models to unfold the roughness properties from the scattering data. This has been done in the second experiment with a set of six sinusoidal surfaces with varying amplitudes and spatial periods [9]. The data for these surfaces consist of a set of sharp diffraction peaks as shown in Figure 7. To measure this sharply peaked angular distribution, the DALLAS instrument was used in a special high resolution mode with a single scanning detector, whose angular scanning is obtained by rotating the yoke. The profiles for these surfaces were modeled as a

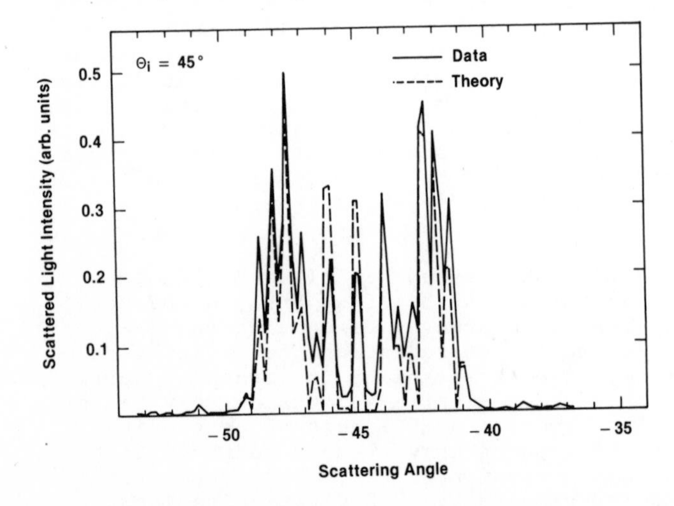

Figure 7. Scattering from an approximately sinusoidal surface ruled in nickel. The rms amplitude is 0.3 μm and the spatial period is 101 μm. $\theta_i = 45°$ is the angle of incidence (from Reference 9).

simple sine wave with two unknown parameters, amplitude (A) and spatial period (D). As in the previous experiments, the scattering from this profile model with assumed values for A and D are calculated, and the resulting angular scattering distribution is compared with the data. Then a search is made for the values of A and D that yield a best fit between the data and the theory. The best values for A are converted to the roughness average R_a which is the average absolute deviation of the profile about the mean line. R_a is a commonly used parameter in surface metrology [5]. Although for a periodic surface the spacing D is simply predictable from the spacing of the diffraction peaks, the amplitude is not so simply obtained. However, for a given D, it appears that A is related to the overall width of the scattering distribution.

These optical measurements of R_a and D are compared in Table 1 with those measured by the stylus technique. The results are uniformly excellent and are well within the uncertainty estimates for these techniques. In the case of the Brass 3 surface, the diffraction peaks were too close to be adequately resolved by the angular scattering instrument. For this surface, a value for D of 800 μm was assumed and the ensuing search yielded a best value for R_a of 1.00 μm in excellent agreement with the value measured by stylus.

Table 1. Inverse scattering calculations for sinusoidal surfaces to derive amplitude (R_a in μm) and wavelength (D in μm).

	measured by stylus		deduced from optical scattering	
	R_a	D	R_a	D
Brass 1	1.02	40.1	1.02	39.9
Brass 2	1.02	100.2	1.01	99.6
Brass 3	1.01	800	1.00	(800)
Nickel 1	1.03	100.2	1.01	100.2
Nickel 2	0.31	100.2	0.31	100.8
Nickel 3	2.98	100.1	2.99	99.3

Thus far, the direct scattering for random surfaces with a dominant lay pattern and the inverse scattering for sinusoidal surfaces have been studied. Future research will involve basically two areas. One is the direct scattering for surfaces with random roughness in both directions. The other is the inverse scattering for random rough surfaces with a dominant lay to obtain parameters such as rms roughness and autocorrelation length. The general inverse scattering problem for arbitrarily rough surfaces is far more difficult and requires detailed studies of the computational techniques.

Characterization of defects

Optical scanning techniques are widely used to detect the presence of defects on surfaces. In a typical situation, a laser beam is scanned over the surface of moving material, and a defect is observed as a change in the scattered laser light. The defect shape is much more difficult to quantify from scattered light measurements, although, in principle, it should be possible to obtain such parameters as the width and depth of the defect.

Experiments have been performed on infrared scattering from carefully measured grooves to study the relationship between the groove shape and the angular scattering distribution and to test the predictions from a rigorous light scattering theory [10,11]. In one of these experiments, the grooves were carefully manufactured to approximate a V-shape and then measured by a precise stylus profiling instrument. The scattering measurements were performed with a CO_2 laser (wavelength 10.53 μm). To calculate light scattering from fairly arbitrary groove shapes, including the resonance region where groove dimensions are of the order of the wavelength, a vector theory was used [12]. The only assumptions and requirements were (1) that the surface be a perfect conductor, (2) that the incoming radiation have transverse electric (TE) polarization, (3) that the topography of the groove be a function of only one direction on the surface and be smooth in the perpendicular direction (Figure 8), and (4) that the width of the groove be less than 10 μm. The last restriction is imposed only due to computer size and time restrictions. Apart from these restrictions, grooves of fairly arbitrary shape can be handled rigorously. Their profiles were digitized and substituted into the theoretical calculation to yield a theoretical angular scattering distribution.

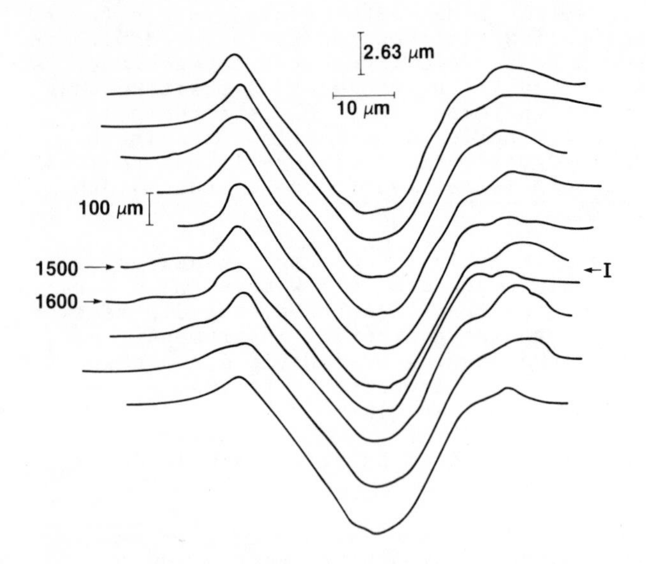

Figure 8. Diamond profilometer measurements of the V-grooves scribed by a diamond on a brass block after the block was polished to an optical surface. Profiles are 100 μm apart. Profiles at 1500 and 1600 μm from the end are used for calculating spectra (from Reference 11).

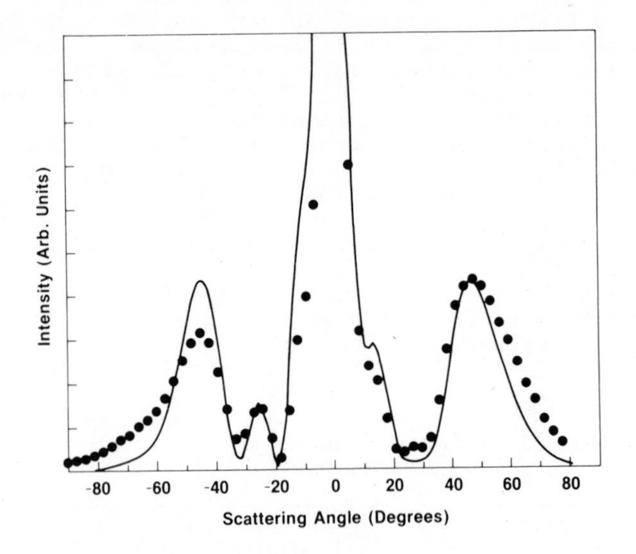

Figure 9. Composite scattering observed at site I (see Figure 8), dots, and scattering computed from a linear combination of the profiles at 1500 and 1600 μm, line (from Reference 11).

Figure 9 shows one of the results comparing the angular scattering data with the calculation. The measured points (solid dots) agree very well with the shape of the theoretical curve. In particular, the agreement in peak position is very good and the overall agreement in intensity is good. The angular scattering distribution is sensitive not only to the depth and width of the groove but to details such as its asymmetry. Figure 8 shows the set of stylus profiles that were used as the source data for the theoretical scattering calculations. In particular, the two profiles adjacent to position I, labeled as 1500 and 1600, were used as the source of data for Figure 8. This averaging, which improved agreement between theory and experiment, was done to take into account about a 100 μm uncertainty in beam position. The diameter of the laser spot was approximately 100 μm.

This work is a step toward the realization of an NDE technique for the quantitative measurement of the geometry of scratch-like defects on surfaces.

Scratch standards

The most important (qualitative) descriptor of optical surface quality used in the United States is the Scratch and Dig Standard (MIL-O-13830A). The characterization of digs (a roughly circular gouge) is fairly well understood, but the characterization of scratches has had a history of technical difficulties [13,14]. Classification of the scratches depends on evaluation by qualified inspectors. Typically, the inspector visually compares the light scattered by an unknown scratch with that scattered by a set of secondary standards scribed in glass with scratch numbers of 10, 20, 40, 60, and 80. The #10 scratch is the mildest defect and scatters the least amount of light, and the #80 scratch is the most serious defect.

Calibration problems arise partly because these scratch numbers do not bear a direct relationship to geometrical parameters such as scratch width. In addition, there is a potential problem that the primary standards upon which this measurment system is based may have changed in respect to their geometrical and light scattering properties since the mid 1940s when the Scratch and Dig Standard was developed. Moreover, the secondary standards, which are sent into the field, are difficult to manufacture reproducibly. To solve these problems, NBS is collaborating in the development of a new set of artifact standards whose light scattering properties will match existing ones but which will have well characterized geometries.

This proposal calls for a set of gratings with rectangular grooves etched on glass. The width, depth, spacing, and total number of the grooves are controlled to produce the appropriate light scattering characteristics. In addition, the spacings between the grooves are modulated (or "chirped") to generate a broad scattering pattern with a peak slightly off the axis of the illuminating beam. In general, the designs call for gratings having on the order of 10 grooves with depths of about one wavelength of visible light and widths of about 1 to 1.5 μm. Some of the prototype groove artifacts were chemically etched in glass, whereas others were etched by an ion-beam.

Figure 10 compares the scattering results for several of these new prototypes with results from an existing set of scratch standards. It shows graphs of relative scattered

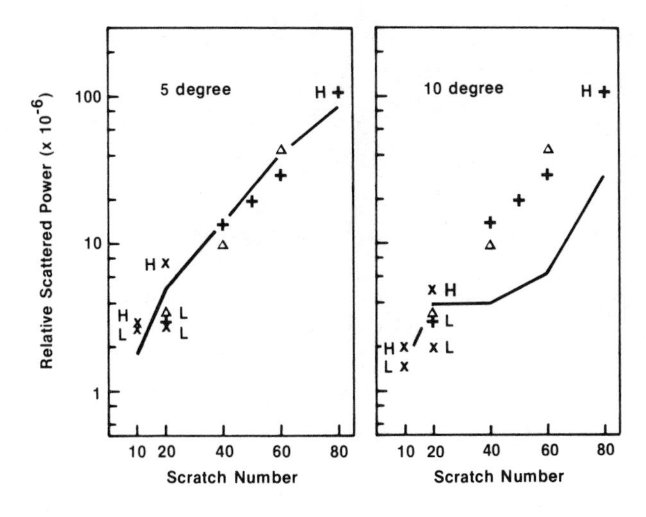

Figure 10. Power scattered by etched glass artifacts at ± 5° and ± 10°, as a function of scratch number determined by visual comparison with secondary standards. The scattering due to existing secondary scratch standards is plotted as the solid line. The scattering due to new prototype standards is represented by the points X, +, and Δ and designated H or L. These symbols are described in the text (from Reference 14).

light intensity measured at scattering angles of 5 and 10 degrees, respectively, as a function of the scratch number. Average scattering by the existing secondary standards is plotted as the solid line, and the values due to the various new prototypes are plotted as the various points (+, X, and Δ). H or L means, for example, that by visual comparison with the primary scratch standards the new prototype was designated, respectively, as a high or low #10 or #20, as the case may be. The peak power scattered by the prototypes as a function of their scratch number falls quite close to the 5° data represented by the solid line (Figure 10, left), obtained with existing secondary standards. Thus, the etched prototypes, which should lend themselves to reproducible manufacturing, can be used in place of the existing, scribed, secondary standards under these experimental conditions.

Although more development work needs to be done, the proposed new scratch artifacts hold promise as standards whose geometries, and therefore scattering properties, can be well characterized. It may be noted, however, that this work is aimed at standardizing what is observed visually from surfaces containing scratches, whereas the work on scattering previously discussed [10,11] was aimed at a quantitative evaluation of the geometry of surface imperfections.

4. Optical microscopy

Linewidth and other critical dimensions on integrated-circuit (IC) wafers and photomasks must be known and accurately controlled to enable IC performance to be predicted from design specifications, to facilitate transfer of accurate photomask dimensions between manufacturer and user, and to monitor lithographic and patterning processes during microchip manufacture. The most widely used instruments for making linewidth measurements on photomasks and wafers have been based on optical imaging, i.e., those employing a microscope in conjunction with some type of measuring attachment. Traditional measurement systems have not been able to achieve the accuracy and precision at micrometer and submicrometer dimensions required for VLSI geometries.

The accuracy of optical imaging methods is dependent upon the characteristics of the optical image formed by the microscope and is affected by diffraction and aberrations in the optical systems, as well as the coherence of the illumination. As shown in Figure 11, even with very steep material edges, the optical image contains a gradual transition from light to dark at the line edge. The width of the transition region or image edge is comparable to the diameter of the diffraction spot, or Airy disk, of the imaging optics, and is approximately 1 μm for a 0.65 numerical aperture (N.A.). To determine linewidth to an accuracy better than this, an optical threshold or other criterion based on a theoretical model that yields the true edge location must be used.

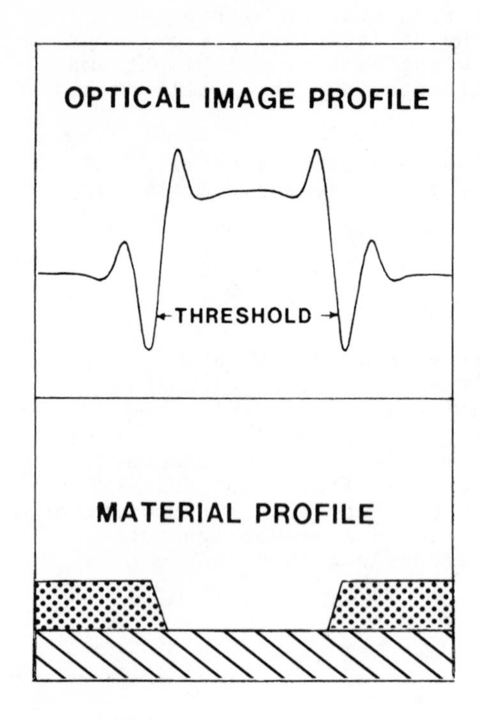

Figure 11. Schematic representation of the relationship between the material edges and the optical image.

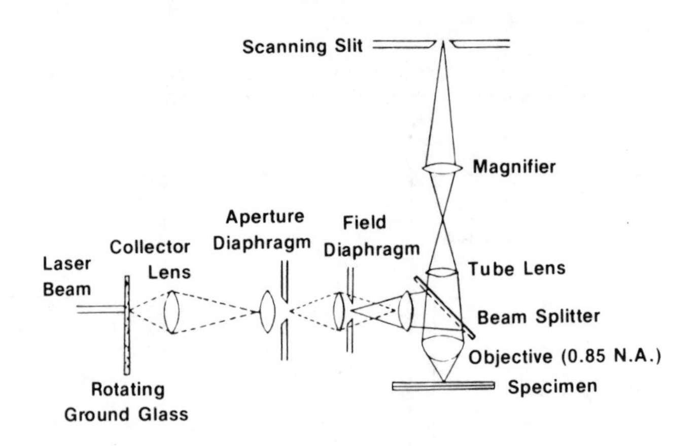

Figure 12. Ray path for a reflected-light, laser microscope system (from Reference 15).

Although linewidth measurements on photomasks may be made with either transmitted or reflected light, transmitted light is preferred because of the lower sensitivity to variations in edge geometry, film thickness variations, and surface contamination. Silicon wafers, of course, must be measured in reflected light. In all cases, an effectively spatially coherent imaging system is desirable to avoid degradation of the edge response. For wafers viewed in reflected light, the optical parameters of reflectance and phase are strongly dependent on both wavelength and angle of incidence. Therefore, these parameters are uniquely defined only for a single wavelength (or narrow spectral bandwith) and angle of incidence. Thus, a more highly coherent imaging system characterized by a narrow cone angle of illumination and narrower spectral bandwidth is required for wafer measurements.

A primary linewidth measurement system using a laser source with a reflected light imaging system has been developed at NBS [15]. This system, shown schematically in Figure 12, may be described as a modified bright-field, image-scanning microscope. The illumination source is a 1 W krypton (530 nm) or argon (514 nm) ion laser. A rotating ground-glass disk is used to reduce and control the spatial coherence of the laser beam, which would otherwise produce undesirable speckle and interference effects. The system has a linewidth measurement precision (three sigma) of approximately 0.04 μm for linewidth and line-spacing dimensions from 0.5 to 10 μm. The entire system is mounted on a vibration-isolation table in a temperature-controlled environment (22 ± 1 °C). In addition, the NBS system is sufficiently versatile as a research tool to allow variations in light sources and other optical system parameters.

For thin, patterned layers, i.e., less than $\lambda/4$ thick, where λ is the wavelength of light, a scalar coherence theory of imaging in the microscope has been used; it assumes that the characteristics of the sample (line object) can be described by a 1-D complex reflectance function that varies in the direction of scan. Specifically, it is assumed that the object consists of a discontinuous change in reflectance as well as a discontinuous change in the optical phase introduced at the line edge on reflection (or transmission). A comparison between the image profile predicted by this theory and the image profile obtained with the NBS linewidth-measuring system is shown in Figure 13, which shows the very good accuracy that can be achieved [16]. However, in addition to the theoretical image dependence upon the assumptions of monochromatic illumination and a prescribed degree of spatial coherence, this model and the coherent edge detection threshold require knowledge of the phase difference introduced at the line edge by radiation reflected from the two materials, i.e., here silicon dioxide and silicon. This phase difference occurs due to the difference in phase change on reflection from different materials as well as the path

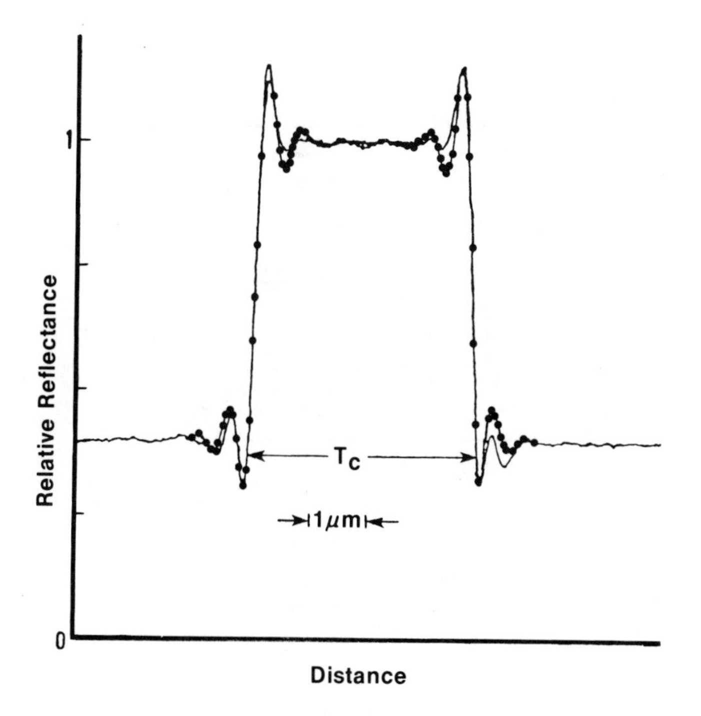

Figure 13. Comparison of experimental (—) and theoretical (—•—•—) image profiles for a window etched in a 150-nm thick layer of silicon dioxide on silicon (0.85 objective N.A., 0.2 condenser N.A., and 530 nm wavelength). T_c is the optical threshold at the line edge (from Reference 16).

difference at the line edge and is, therefore, sensitive to variations in the thickness and index of refraction of the patterned layer and sublayers. To circumvent the requirement for accurate knowledge of this phase difference, a dual-threshold, edge-detection and focusing criterion has been developed [17] based on scalar image theory. Thus, when the phase difference is unknown and varies with normal processing, the dual threshold method is the superior method.

Although scalar theory can be used to describe scattering from a limited range of objects such as photomasks or thin layers of oxide or nitride on silicon, for features thicker than approximately $\lambda/4$, this theory of partially coherent (spatial) imaging breaks down. Unfortunately, most of the features including resist and metal lines, which need to be measured during the production of IC microchips fall into this category of thick objects. To deal with this important case, a monochromatic waveguide model has been developed that can predict the optical microscope images of thick-layer objects, including those whose index of refraction and geometry vary with depth in the layer [16,18,19]. A representation of a cross section of a line patterned in a thick layer and the corresponding multilayer representation is shown in Figure 14.

In order to test this model, a specimen was prepared consisting of lines patterned in photoresist on a silicon substrate. Two patterns were selected to illustrate different edge properties: one with nearly vertical edge walls; and the second with significantly sloping edges. Figure 15 compares the experimental and theoretical image profiles produced by these structures. Since "best" focus has not been adequately defined for imaging of thick structures, a series of profiles corresponding to varying focal positions have been obtained. The results for two focal positions are illustrated in Figure 15 and compared with the theoretical data. The image profile is very sensitive to edge geometry, and without an accurate model the exact locations of the line edges cannot be determined. Although the theoretical and experimental profiles display the same features, the agreement is certainly not perfect. Some possible sources of error include inhomogeneity in the resist; variations in edge geometry along the length of the line; illumination in the microscope that subtends a finite cone angle, whereas the waveguide model treats the scattered field at normal incidence only; and possible asymmetry in the illumination in the microscope. Although the alignment of the measurement system was checked for illumination symmetry for profiling thin layers, it is expected that thick layers such as the resist used here are significantly more sensitive to asymmetric illumination than are thin-layer objects and, therefore, may require tighter alignment tolerances.

The waveguide model described here is currently being applied to other materials including metals and multi-layer features as well as the development of focus criteria and algorithms for determination of linewidth and feature geometry. This model also enables the relationship between process variations in the materials and resulting image profile to be determined and this, in turn, enables the accuracy and sensitivity of different measurement techniques to be investigated. However, to improve the accuracy and repeatability of

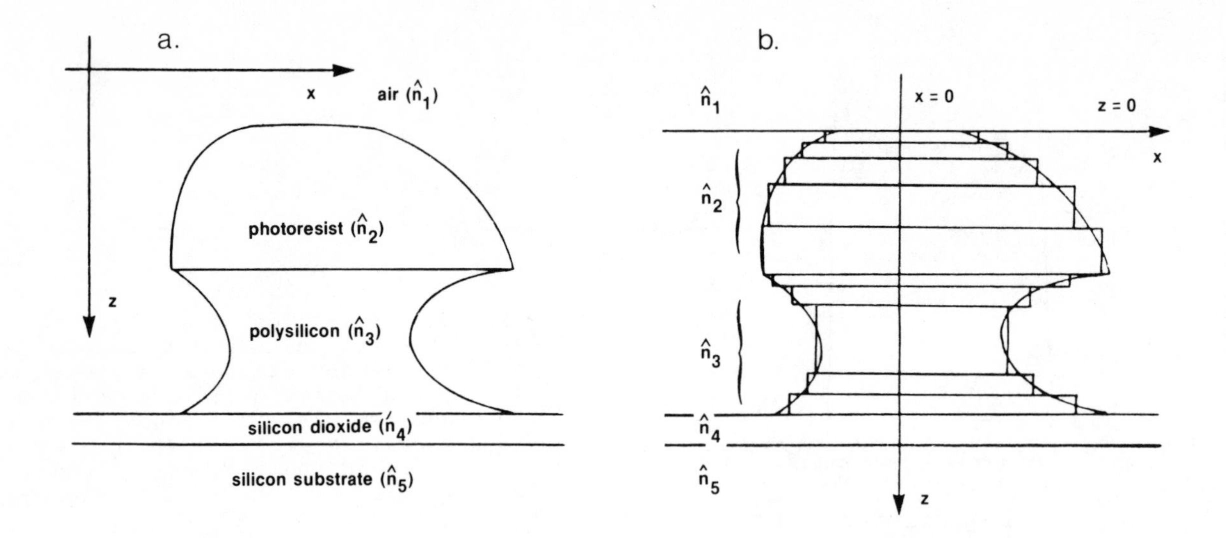

Figure 14. Cross section of a representative line object (a) and the corresponding multilayer representation (b). $\hat{n}$ is the complex index of refraction, z is the optical axis, and x is the direction of scan.

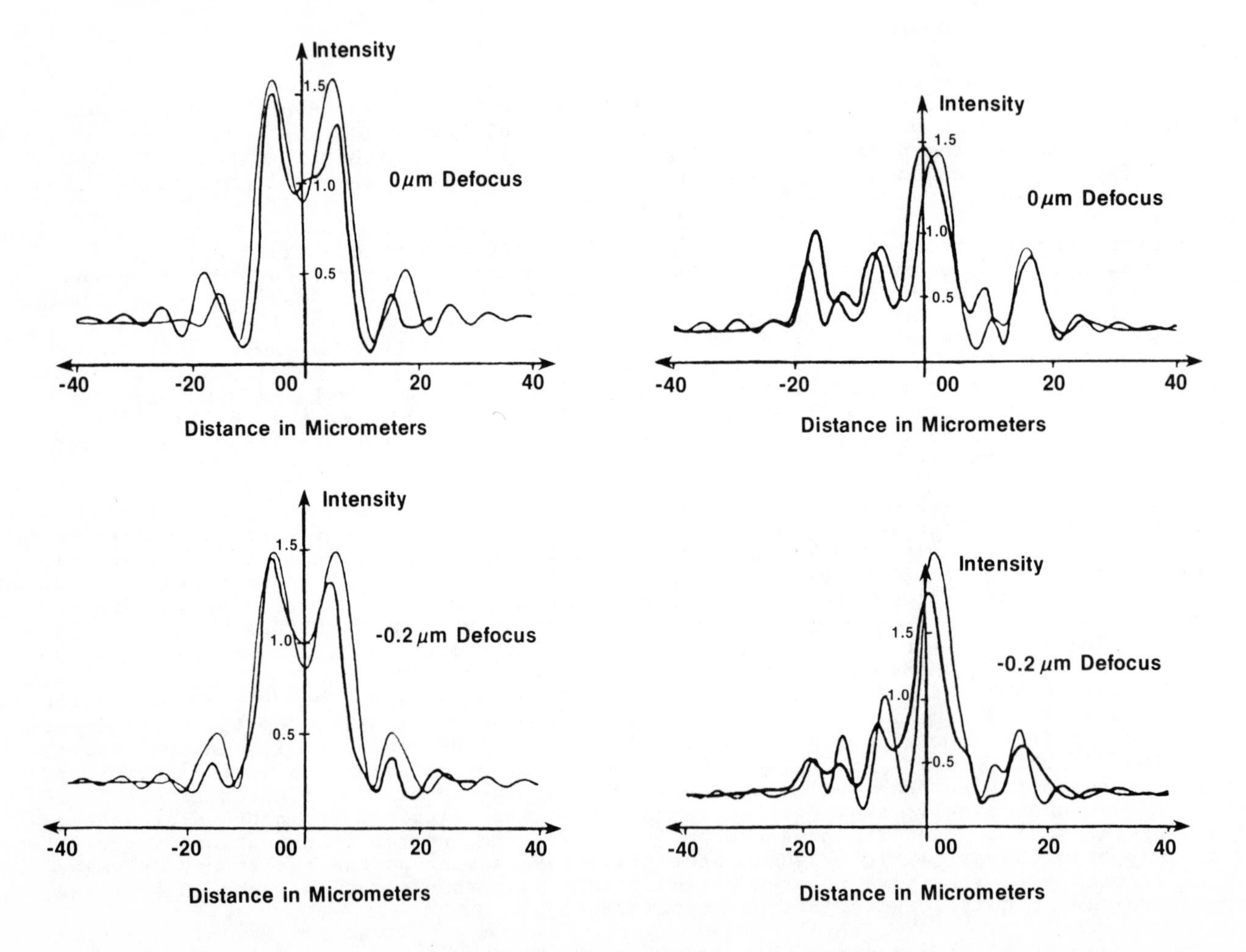

Figure 15. Comparison of experimental and theoretical image intensity profiles of a window in photoresist on silicon. The window has either vertical edge walls (left) or sloping edge walls (right). The experimental profiles are shown by the thick line and the theoretical profiles by the thin line. The photoresist was assumed to have a thickness of 0.94 μm (from Reference 19).

linewidth measurements made during IC manufacture, more work is needed on the development of measurement techniques which yield the geometrical parameters of the line independent of process variations in the materials (index of refraction, thickness, etc.).

The optical microscope outlined here is a primary linewidth measurement system. NBS currently calibrates with a transmitted light version of this system transfer standards for optical linewidth measurements on photomasks (standard reference materials (SRMs) 474, 475, and 476) and is currently developing such standards for wafers. Because linewidth measurement systems such as those used in the IC industry typically use a fixed edge-detection criterion and are, therefore, unable to correct for differences in materials, the optical parameters of the transfer standard used for calibration must match those of the part to be measured. When they do not match, calibration errors result and go undetected through the calibration and measurement process.

5. Scattering from particles

As shown in Section 3, the development of laser scattering techniques has facilitated the quantitative characterization of surface topography. In addition, such techniques have facilitated the nonintrusive measurements of flowing particles, which have been used for combustion diagnostics and should be useful in sensing actual combustion systems. The spatial distribution of mean particle size and particle number concentration can be obtained from measurements of the scattered light by using highly focused laser beams [20,21]. It is also possible to determine the spatial distribution of particle volume fraction for absorbing particles from measurements of the extinction coefficient, although this transmittance is the integrated value of the local extinction coefficient along the optical path. To obtain the local values, it is necessary to employ an inversion technique which is widely used in tomographic reconstruction [22]. In addition, laser Doppler velocimetry can be employed to measure the axial, radial, and tangential velocity components of droplets [23]. An experimental arrangement for such particle-sizing and velocity measurements is shown in Figure 16.

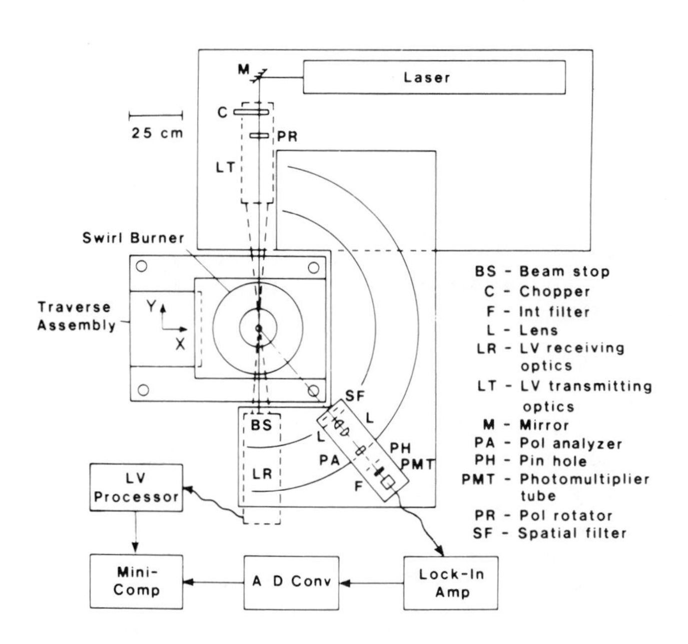

Figure 16. Schematic of laser scattering apparatus for determining droplet size, number density, and velocity. Traverse assembly is used for moving the swirl burner in combustion spray studies to probe the droplet properties in the measurement volume. Applications to other physical systems are made by removing the burner. The dual-beam laser velocimeter is represented by the dashed lines; the intersecting dashed lines represent two laser beams (from Reference 20).

Such methods have been applied to study the combustion of sprays, a complicated phenomenon which involves the interaction of complex physical and chemical processes. The combustion of liquid fuel sprays is central to the operation of a wide variety of practical combustion systems such as industrial furnaces and boilers, gas turbines and direct injection engines, and other liquid fuel fired power systems. The ability to improve combustion efficiency and to predict and ultimately control pollutant formation in fuel spray flames requires the type of detailed information that can be obtained by the light scattering measurements mentioned above. Although these techniques have been developed for application to combustion diagnostics, they should find application in monitoring and controlling processes involving flowing particles, in general, because they are noninvasive and do not disturb the medium being studied. As an example of the application of such techniques extended to opaque particles, consider a program which has been recently initiated at NBS to study the processing of rapidly solidified metal powders and to develop sensors based on these techniques for monitoring the process. The unique benefits of rapid solidification may be attained only if the particles are solidified under certain specific conditions which require, among other things, knowledge of droplet size, distribution, and velocity. In addition to the previously developed methods for measuring such quantities, a major component of this program is a high-pressure, inert gas, atomization unit capable of 23-kg batch runs, which has recently become operational. Figure 17 illustrates this unit and the possible location of real-time light scattering sensors to provide data for monitoring the production of solidified metal powders.

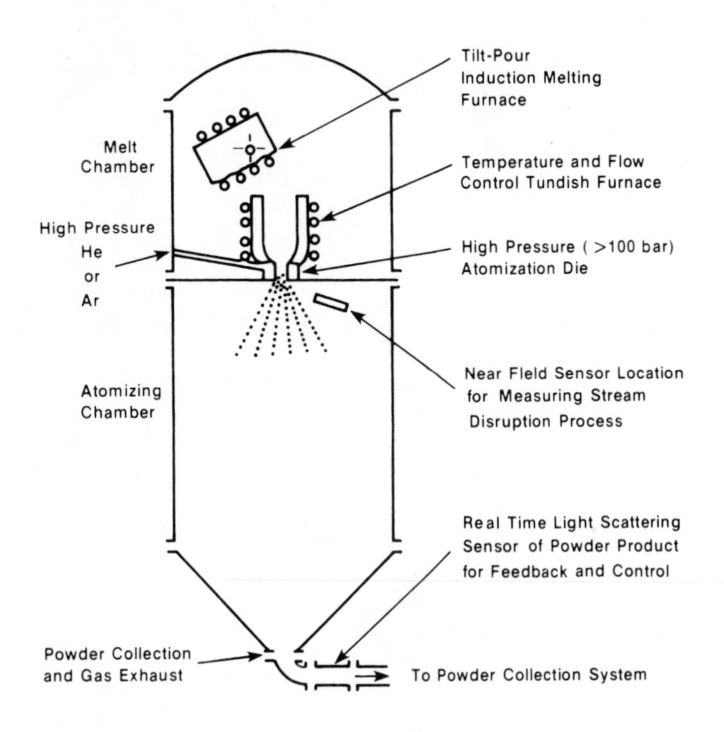

Figure 17. NBS high pressure inert gas atomizer for the rapid solidification of metal powders, illustrating proposed arrangement for metal powder diagnostics.

In order to more fully quantify the light-scattering properties of the metal particles, detailed Mie scattering calculations are being undertaken. Similar calculations carried out for particles in combustion systems have provided valuable insights for interpreting the optical measurements [24]. The overall objective of this study is to provide a sound scientific data base from which to develop appropriate sensors and control monitoring approaches for rapid solidification processes.

6. Optical fiber techniques

Cure monitoring of polymer matrix composites

Optical fibers are used as light pipes or waveguides to conduct light from a source, usually a laser, to some detector. Their principal use in NDE is as a sensor in which their interaction with their environment resulting from temperature, strain, and acoustic waves, for example, has an effect on the light transmitted through the fiber [25]. A rather different NDE application of optical fibers described here is in the cure monitoring of polymer matrix composites [26,27].

The manufacture of polymer matrix composites involves complicated chemical and physical changes that must be adequately controlled to produce desirable products. The major chemical change that occurs in processing is the transformation from liquid monomer to the solid, cross-linked, polymer matrix. The chemical and physical structure of the polymer matrix/reinforcement interface is thought to have a significant effect on properties and performance. Since the interfacial region between the fiber reinforcement and the resin matrix encompasses an exceedingly small volume of material that is difficult to probe, there is little known about this region. However, since debonding at the interface can adversely affect mechanical properties of composites, it is important to be able to probe this region during processing, particularly, during curing when the resin undergoes a transformation from a liquid to a solid.

This transformation can be followed by the fluorescence spectra of organic dyes dissolved in epoxy resins. These dyes are sensitive to the local viscosity [28], and their concentration is too low to affect the resins. For such dyes, there is a marked change in the fluorescent intensity as the resin changes from its liquid to solid state. The method of monitoring this fluorescence is illustrated in Figure 18 where the fiber reinforcement might be used as the light pipe, or suitable fibers could be introduced into the matrix without significantly altering the mechanical properties of the composite. The evanescent wave of the laser light, i.e., the light field extending beyond the fiber, probes the material surrounding the fiber to a depth that depends on the refractive indices of the fiber and matrix (resin). A probe molecule in the vicinity of the fiber will be excited by this evanescent wave, and its emission may be viewed in several ways; at right angles to the fiber direction, at the end of a neighboring fiber, or at either end of the propagating fiber. Monitoring the fluorescence then provides a means of determining the changes in microviscosity, averaged along the length of the fiber, near the fiber-matrix interface as curing proceeds. The results obtained thus far towards implementing the procedure illustrated in Figure 18 are encouraging. Preliminary experiments have shown that one part of the fluorescence spectrum of an excimer forming dye is sensitive to viscosity, while another part that is not sensitive to viscosity serves as an internal standard.

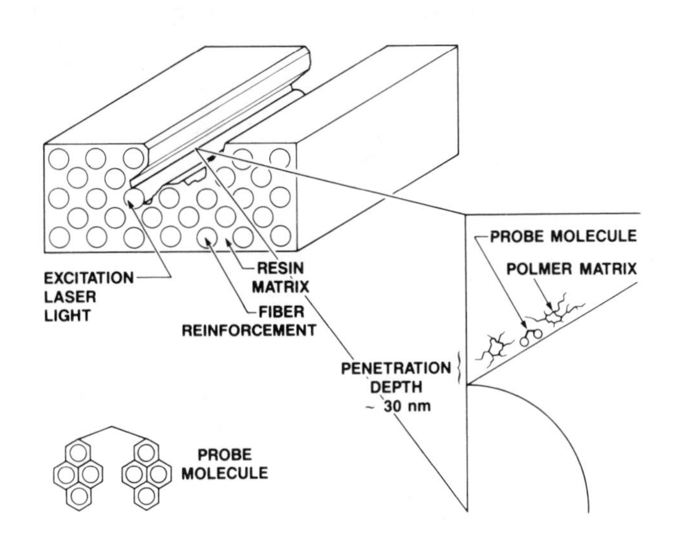

Figure 18. Schematic representation of the experimental approach to on-line process monitoring of the curing of polymer matrix composites, using optical waveguides (fibers) and a fluorescent probe (from Reference 26).

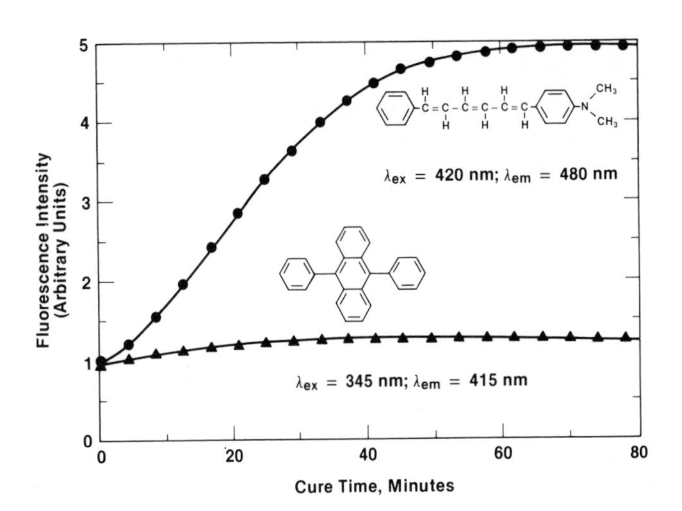

Figure 19. Fluorescence intensities as a function of cure time of the viscosity sensitive dye (DMA-DPH) at 480 nm (dots) and of the viscosity insensitive dye (DPA) at 415 nm (triangles) (from Reference 27).

Unfortunately, the excimer forming dyes are insensitive to the higher viscosities that must be sensed, that is, viscosities beyond the gel point. However, other dye systems have been found that are sensitive to viscosity changes in the gel to glass-solid range. These dyes do not have internal fluorescence standards and thereby require the introduction of a second dye whose fluorescence intensity is insensitive to local viscosity. The result of this procedure is illustrated in Figure 19. This figure shows the fluorescent intensity as a function of cure time when laser excitation at 420 nm and 345 nm is used to produce fluorescence, respectively, at 480 nm from the viscosity-sensitive dye and fluorescence at 415 nm from the viscosity-insensitive dye. The fluorescent intensity of the former increased with cure time while that of the latter remained practically constant. The intensity ratio increased steadily with cure time and reached a plateau at the end of the cure. This intensity ratio is not sensitive to the geometry of the sample, light intensity, and optical input and output coupling arrangement. It therefore monitors the cure of samples which contain reinforcing fibers and has the potential for being adopted to in situ monitoring of the cure of composite structures in the factory environment.

Determination of fiber fracture

It was mentioned earlier that optical fibers have potential as strain measuring elements. Since this element can be incorporated within the structure of composite materials without any noticeable deterioration in their mechanical properties, there appears to be considerable potential for this technique both for NDE and for continuous in-service monitoring of the stress history of a composite [25]. It may be possible to use the same fibers for more than one NDE purpose, e.g., cure monitoring and strain gauging. In any case, a novel approach may be mentioned to measure fiber fracture in composites, an important NDE measurement, since fracture of fiber-reinforced composites may begin as a single fiber fracture [29]. With optical fibers substituted for the conventional reinforcement in a woven composite, the crack opening displacement (COD) between broken fiber ends has been measured in the 5 to 90 μm range. This has been accomplished by measuring with a He-Ne laser a $1/R^2$ decrease in transmitted light intensity with increasing COD, where R is the COD, provided R is greater than roughly 5 μm [29]. This range of COD is of primary concern for engineering materials studies. It is hoped that with such a technique, COD can be measured in situ, which will contribute to a better understanding of the fracture process in composites and may lead to a useful NDE method.

7. Concluding remarks

This review discusses a large variety of optical NDE methods that are being developed and used at the NBS to solve many NDE problems. Some of this work, particularly, the characterization of surface roughness and the accurate measurement of linewidths on wafers and masks is aimed, in part, at developing reference measurement methods and standards. Other work, which includes the study and development of light scattering sensors to monitor the production of rapidly solidified metal powders and the use of optical fibers to follow the curing of polymer matrix composites, is aimed at studying prototype systems for use in the noninvasive monitoring of manufacturing processes. Almost all of the work described here is a continuing effort, and some of it is in its earliest stages. Nevertheless, the results obtained at this point are encouraging and support the general optimism in the employment of optical NDE techniques for quantitative results and for use in monitoring manufacturing processes.

The authors thank Drs. B. M. Fanconi, D. E. Gilsinn, R. D. Kriz, L. Mordfin, R. J. Santoro, and M. Young for many helpful suggestions, and Dr. S. D. Ridder for Figure 17.

8. References

1. Birnbaum, G., and White, G. S., "Laser Techniques in NDE," Research Techniques in Nondestructive Testing, Vol. VII, edited by R. S. Sharpe, Academic Press, New York, pp. 259-265. 1984.

2. Birnbaum, G., White, G. S., and Vest, C. M., "Laser Generated and Detected Ultrasound and Holographic Methods," Pressure Vessel and Piping Technology 1985--A Decade of Progress, edited by C. Sundararajan, American Society of Mechanical Engineers, New York, Vol. 6.6, pp. 661-669. 1985.

3. Youren, X., Vest, C. M., and Delp, E. J., "Digital and Optical Moiré Detection of Flaws Applied to Holographic Nondestructive Testing," Opt. Letters, Vol. 8, pp. 452-454. 1983.

4. Youren, X., and Vest, C. M., "Holographic Technique for Simultaneous Measurement of Displacement and Tilt," Appl. Opt., Vol. 22, pp. 2137-2140. 1983.

5. Surface Texture, ANSI B46.1-1978, American Society of Mechanical Engineers, New York. 1978.

6. Vorburger, T. V., and Teague, E. C., "Optical Techniques for On-line Measurement of Surface Topography," Prec. Eng., Vol. 3, pp. 61-83. 1981.

7. Church, E. L., Jenkinson, H. A., and Zavada, J. M., "Measurement of the Finish of Diamond-Turned Metal Surfaces by Differential Light Scattering," Opt. Eng., Vol. 16, pp. 360-374. 1977.

8. Vorburger, T. V., Teague, E. C., Scire, F. E., McLay, M. J., and Gilsinn, D. E., "Surface Roughness Studies with DALLAS--Detector Array for Laser Light Angular Scattering," J. Res. NBS, Vol. 89, pp. 3-16. 1984.

9. Vorburger, T. V., Gilsinn, D. E., Scire, F. E., McLay, M. J., Giauque, C. H. W., and Teague, E. C., "Optical Measurement of the Roughness of Sinusoidal Surfaces," Proceedings of the Third International Conference on the Metrology and Properties of Engineering Surfaces, edited by K. J. Stout and T. R. Thomas, Elsevier Sequoia, S. A., Lausanne. 1986.

10. White, G. S., and Feldman, A., "Diffraction from a Shallow Groove," Appl. Opt., Vol. 20, pp. 2585-2589. 1981.

11. White, G. S., and Marchiando, J. F., "Scattering from a V-Shaped Groove in the Resonance Domain," Appl. Opt., Vol. 22, pp. 2308-2312. 1983.

12. Maystre, D., "Electromagnetic Scattering from Perfectly Conducting Rough Surfaces in the Resonance Region," IEEE Trans. Ant. and Prop., Vol. AP-31, pp. 885-895. 1983.

13. Young, M., Johnson, E. G., Jr., and Goldgraben, R., "Tunable Scratch Standards," Proc. SPIE, Vol. 525, pp. 70-77. 1985.

14. Young, M., "Scratch Standard Revisited," to be published.

15. Bullis, W. M., and Nyyssonen, D., "Optical Linewidth Measurements on Photomasks and Wafers," in VLSI Electronics: Microstructure Science, Vol. 3, edited by N. G. Einspruch, Academic Press, New York, pp. 301-346. 1982.

16. Nyyssonen, D., "Theory of Optical Edge Detection and Imaging of Thick Layers," J. Opt. Soc. Am., Vol. 72, pp. 1425-1436. 1982.

17. Nyyssonen, D., "A Practical Method for Edge Detection and Focusing for Linewidth Measurements on Wafers," Proc. SPIE, Vol. 538, pp. 172-178. 1985.

18. Nyyssonen, D., "Optical Linewidth Measurement on Patterned Metal Layers," Proc. SPIE, Vol. 480, pp. 65-70. 1984.

19. Kirk, C. P., and Nyyssonen, D., "Modeling the Optical Microscope Images of Thick Layers for the Purpose of Linewidth Measurement," Proc. SPIE, Vol. 538, pp. 179-187. 1985.

20. Presser, C., Gupta, A. K., Santoro, R. J., and Semerjian, H. G., "Droplet Size Measurements in a Swirling Kerosene Spray Flame by Laser Light Scattering," Proc. International Conference on Liquid Atomization and Spray Systems (ICLASS-85), pp. VIIC/2/1-13. 1985.

21. Santoro, R. J., Semerjian, H. G., and Dobbins, R. A., "Soot Particle Measurements in Diffusion Flames," Combust. and Flame, Vol. 51, pp. 203-218. 1983.

22. Ray, S. R., and Semerjian, H. G., "Laser Tomography for Simultaneous Concentration and Temperature Measurement in Reacting Flows," in Combustion Diagnostics by Nonintrusive Methods, edited by T. D. McCay and J. A. Roux, Progress in Astronautics and Aeronautics, Vol. 92, AIAA, New York, pp. 300-324. 1983.

23. Presser, C., Gupta, A. K., Santoro, R. J., and Semerjian, H. G., "Velocity and Droplet Size Measurements in a Fuel Spray," Paper No. AIAA-86-0297 at the AIAA 24th Aerospace Sciences Meeting, Reno, Nevada. 1986.

24. Dobbins, R. A., Santoro, R. J., and Semerjian, H. G., "Interpretation of Optical Measurements of Soot in Flames," in Combustion Diagnostics by Nonintrusive Methods, edited by T. D. McCay and J. A. Roux, Progress in Astronautics and Aeronautics, Vol. 92, pp. 208-237. 1984.

25. Culshaw, B., "Fiber Optic Sensing Techniques," in Research Techniques in NDT, Vol. 7, edited by R. S. Sharpe, Academic Press, pp. 192-215. 1984.

26. Fanconi, B. M., Wang., F. W., Hunston, D., and Mopsik, F., "Cure Monitoring for Polymer Matrix Composites," Materials Characterization for Systems Performance and Reliability, edited by J. W. McCauley and V. Weiss, Plenum Pub. Corp., pp. 275-291. 1986.

27. Wang, F. W., Lowry, R. E., Wu En-Shinn, and Fanconi, B. M., "Fluorescence Methods for Cure Monitoring of Epoxy Resins," Proceedings of Scientific Conference on Chemical Research, Aberdeen Proving Ground. 1985.

28. Oster, G., and Nishijima, Y., "Fluorescence and Internal Rotation: Their Dependence on Viscosity of the Medium," J. Am. Chem. Soc., Vol. 78, pp. 1581-1584. 1956.

29. Kriz, R. D., personal communication.

Shearography versus Holography in Nondestructive Evaluation

Y.Y. Hung

Department of Mechanical Engineering, Oakland University
Rochester, Michigan 48063

Introduction

The demands for greater product quality and product reliability has created a need for better techniques of nondestructive evaluation. Each of the available techniques including ultrasonic, acoustical emissions, radiography, thermography, magnetic particles, eddy current, dye penetrant, and optical methods such as holography and shearography has its unique advantages and disadvantages. The selection of one technique depends on the particular objective of the evaluation. When selecting a technique, it is important to have a sound knowledge of the capabilities as well as limitations of each technique. This paper will give a thorough review of two major optical methods of nondestructive testing: holography and shearography.

Principles of Holography

Holography is known as three-dimensional photography. However, it is radically different from photography. It does not require the use of lenses or other imaging device but requires coherent light, as from a laser. Holography records a three-dimensional image (wavefront) by means of interference. A laser is needed because light emitting from a laser possesses the ability of destructive and constructive interference. Holography allows the wavefronts of an object to be recorded and subsequently displayed three-dimensionally in space. One of the most important applications of holography in engineering is hologram interferometry which allows an object to be compared with itself in a slightly deformed state. Holographic nondestructive evaluation employs hologram interferometry.

Figure 1 shows a typical optical arrangement for holographic nondestructive evaluation. The laser beam is expanded and illuminates the object being evaluated. A small portion of the expanded beam is reflected by the mirror M1 to the convexed mirror M2 which further expands the beam and directs it onto a high-resolution recording medium such as a photographic plate. The light scattered from the object meets reference beam producing an interference pattern which is recorded by the photographic plate. The processed photography on which a three dimensional image of the object is stored is known as a hologram. The three-dimensional image is coded in dense interference patterns in the plate. To decode, the hologram is illuminated with a reconstruction beam as shown in Figure 2. The hologram diffracts the reconstruction wave in such a way that a three-dimensional image of the object is displayed in space. It is a truely three-dimensional image as it possesses depth, parallax and other properties associated with real objects.

Hologram interferometry is based on the interference of two overlapping images. Because the images do not contain mass, two three-dimensional images can be overlapped and compared. The two overlapped images of the same object interferes with each other producing a fringe pattern which depicts the phase difference between the two wavefronts. This is the basis of hologram interferometry. There are four methods of performing hologram interferometry, namely - double exposure, real-time, sandwich and time-average techniques. Here only the double exposure technique will be used to demonstrate the principles. The double exposure technique utilizes the multiple storage capability of a hologram, i.e. more than one image can be recorded on a single hologram. This allows two images of the same object to be recorded sequentially in a single photographic plate and subsequently displayed simultaneously. The result of the two overlapping images is a interference pattern which depicts surface displacements of the deformation. The interference patterns are generally called fringe patterns.

In nondestructive testing, the photographic plate is doubly exposed: first with the object in the undeformed state, and second, exposure after the object has been deformed. The hologram thus stores two images corresponding to the deformed and undeformed states of the same object. Upon reconstruction, the two images are displayed simultaneously and they may interfere with each other producing a fringe pattern which depicts surface displacement of the object due to the deformation. The fringe pattern is mathematically represented by:

$$I = I_0 (1 + \cos \Delta) \qquad (1)$$

Where $\Delta = \frac{2\pi}{\lambda} (Au + Bv + Cw) \qquad (2)$

A, B and C are sensitivity factors which are give by:

$$A = \frac{x - x_o}{R_o} + \frac{x - x_s}{R_s}$$

$$B = \frac{y - y_o}{R_o} + \frac{y - y_s}{R_s} \qquad (3)$$

$$C = \frac{z - z_o}{R_o} + \frac{z - z_s}{R_s}$$

Where (x_s, y_s, z_s) is the location of the illumination; (x_o, y_o, z_o) is the position of the camera, and $R_o^2 = X_o^2 + Y_o^2 + Z_o^2$, $R_s^2 = X_s^2 + Y_s^2 + Z_s^2$.

Principles of Shearography

Shearography is a laser optical method originally developed for strain measurements. Contrary to holography which measures surface displacements, shearography measures derivatives of surface displacements. Since strains are functions of displacement derivatives, shearography allows strains to be determined without numerically differentiating displacement data. Note that numerical differentiation is laborious and prone to large errors.

The set-up of shearography is illustrated in Figure 3. The object to be measured is illuminated with a point source of coherent light and it is imaged by a image-shearing camera. A photographic film in the image plane is exposed twice with the object being deformed between the exposures. The processed photograph yields a fringe pattern depicting the derivatives of the surface displacements. This fringe pattern is not readily visible on the processed photographic film; it is made visible by a high-pass Fourier filtering process to be described later.

Shearography utilizes a shearing-camera which differs from an ordinary camera in that it is equipped with a shearing device. While various devices and methods may be used to accomplish the shearing effect, only one method is herein described. The shearing device consists of a thin glass wedge located at the iris plane of the lens, and it covers one-half of the camera lens. Without the wedge, rays scattered from an object point, and received by the two halves of the lens will converge to a point in the image; i.e., a point on the object is mapped into a point in the image plane. The wedge is a small angle prism which deviates rays passing through it. In the presence of the wedge, the rays from the object point P are mapped into two points P1 and P2 in the image plane. This is illustrated in Figure 4. Thus, a pair of laterally sheared images is observed in the image plane. In other words, the image-shearing camera brings the rays scattered from one point on the object's surface to interfere with those scattered from a neighboring point. This is illustrated in Figure 5. Since the object is illuminated with coherent light, the rays from the two points interfere producing a random interference pattern (commonly known as a speckle pattern). When the object is deformed, a relative displacement between the two points occurs. This relative displacement produces a relative phase change which slightly modifies the interference speckle pattern. Superposition of these two speckle patterns (deformed and undeformed) produces a beat fringe pattern which depicts the relative displacement between the two neighboring points. If the wedge is so oriented that the rays are deviated in the xz-plane, the shearing is in the x-direction. And if the magnitude of the shearing is small, the fringe pattern of Equation (1) depicts the derivatives of the displacements with respect to x with:

$$\Delta = \frac{2\pi}{\lambda} \left(A\frac{\partial u}{\partial x} + B\frac{\partial v}{\partial x} + C\frac{\partial w}{\partial x}\right) \partial x \qquad (4)$$

Where ∂x is the amount of shearing, and A, B, C are the sensitivity factors of Equation (3). Should the shearing be in the y-direction, the displacement derivatives of the above equation are with respect to y.

Fringe readout:

It should be noted that the beat fringes produced by the superposition of two speckle patterns are of the frequency modulation type. This type of fringe pattern is different from the conventional fringe patterns as it is not readily visible. Coventional fringes are loci at which intensity is minimum, hence are readily visible to the eye. The present fringe pattern are identified as areas of nulling carriers. That is speckles are nulled along fringe lines. However, the average intensity is uniform, hence the fringe pattern is not characterized by intensity variation and are not readily visible. An optical high pass frequency filtering is needed to convert the invisible frequency modulation fringe pattern to a visible intensity variation fringes.

Figure 6 shows a schematic diagram of the optical high-pass filtering setup. A point source of light is focused by the transforming lens (TL) on to a plane known as the frequency plane. The photographic transparency containing a fringe pattern of the frequency variation type is placed at the input plane. The light field appearing in the frequency plane is the Fourier transform of the transmittance of the photographic transparency. The Fourier transform is a transformation from a spatial domain to a frequency domain. In other words, speckles of the various frequencies in the transparency are separated in the frequency plane. The fringe lines (areas of zero frequency) are displayed at the focal point on the optical axis, whereas those of higher frequencies are located off-axis in the frequency plane. By placing an opaque stop on the axis at the frequency plane to block the zero and low frequency components, the contribution from the fringe lines where the speckles are nulled (zero or low frequency) are stopped. When reimaged by the imaging lens (IL) behind the Fourier filtering plane, those areas will appear dark in the image plane (output plane). Thus the filtering process has converted a frequency modulation type fringe pattern to a visible fringe pattern of intensity variation.

How do Shearography and Holography detect flaws

Flaws in materials usually induce strain concentrations when subjected to stress. Holography reveals flaws by identifying flaw-induced displacement anomalies, whereas shearography reveals flaws by looking for flaw-induced strain anomalies. The output of both techniques are fringe patterns. Flaws are identified by the anomalies in the fringe patterns. Although both techniques measure surface deformation, internal flaws can also be detected. This is because internal flaws, unless very remote from the surface, also influence surface deformation, and hence can be detected. Shearography and holography are most suitable for inspecting plate and shell types of structures, because flaws in such objects are usually not too remote from the surface.

Experimental demonstrations

Shereography and holography have been successfully applied to nondestructive evaluation of many engineering components, such as pressure vessels, disbonds in composite materials, honeycomb structures, steel-reinforced concretes, solid rocket propellant, welded joints, adhesive joints, circuit boards, etc. A few examples are given below.

- Cracks in a pressure vessel - Figure 7a shows the fringe pattern of shearography, whereas Figure 7b is the fringe pattern of holography. The cracks are revealed by both techniques. The means of stressing used is internal pressurization.

- Metal/elastomeric adhesive joints - Figure 8 shows an application of shearography and holography to evaluation of metal/elastomeric adhesive joint. Both techniques clearly detect an disbond at the metal/elastomeric interface. The means of stressing is partial vacuum.

- Ply separations in a tire - The use of shearography and holography for evaluating tires has been accepted by the rubber industry. Both techniques are very effective in detecting ply-separations and voids in tires. Figure 9 shows fringe patterns of a steel-belted truck tire. Several separations along the belt edge of the tire are revealed by both techniques. Partial vacuum is used to stress the tire.

- Flaws at various depth - The shearographic fringe patterns of Figure 10 reveal four separations located in a rubber block at the depth of 3, 6, 9, 12 mm from the surface. The separations are of approximately equal size. The block was stressed by partial vacuum to reveal the flaws. It is seen that the one closer to the surface has higher fringe density and vice versa. This can be readily explaned by assuming that deformation of the rubber above a separation is similar to that of a plate subjected to uniform pressure. Then the magnitude of the surface deflection is inversely proportional to the flexural rigidy of the plate which is proportional to the cube of the thickness (depth).

Shearography versus Holography

Shearography and holography are both interferometric methods, and the output of both are fringe patterns. Holography involves wavefront reconstruction, and the fringe pattern of holography is the result of the interference of the deformed and undeformed wavefronts of the same object. The fringe lines depict surface displacements of the object.

Shearography, on the other hand, is a photographic process which does not reconstruct a three-dimensional image. It records a 3-D object on a 2-D format. The image of shearography contains random interference patterns known as speckles. The speckles act as information carriers about the object surface. When the object is deformed, the speckles are modified. The two speckle patterns corresponding to undeformed and deformed object state produce fringe pattern by more phenomenen. The fringe pattern of shearography depicts the derivatives of surface displacements.

Both shearography and holography measure surface deformation. One fundamental difference between the two techniques is the information they yield. Holography yields surface displacement information, whereas shearography yields derivatives of the surface displacements. For comparison purposes, Figure

11 shows a fringe pattern depicting the deflection W of a rectangular plate clamped along its four sides and centrally loaded, and Figure 12 is the corresponding fringe pattern obtained with shearography. Note that the fringe pattern of holography appears as a single concentric fringe whereas the fringe pattern of shearography is a double concentric fringe pattern. To explain the difference, a plot of the deflection W along the center line x - as is shown in Figure 13a and a plot of the corresponding deflection gradients is shown in Figure 13c. Figure 13b shows a sketch of the contour of W and the sketch of the contours of W' is shown in Figure 13d. There are two humps in the displacement derivative plot which explains why a double concentric fringe pattern is formed in shearography.

Shearography seems to be more practical than holography in nondestructive evaluation because it measures strains directly instead of displacements which holography measures. Since flaws normally create strain concentrations, it is easier to correlate flaws with strain anomalies rather than with displacement anomalies. Also rigid body motions do not produce stratin, shearography is insensitive to such motion. Rigid body motions produce confusing, if not misleading fringes in holography. This advantage of shearography is clearly observed in the examples demonstrated. Holography does not reveal the flaws as prominently as shearography because of the background fringes in holography cuased by rigid body motions. Furthermore, holography requires stringent vibration isolation making field applications very difficult. Shearography generally does not require special vibration isolation. Other advantages of shearography over holography are summarized as follows:

° It requires a very simple optical setup, thus eliminating the optical alignment problem.

° The coherent length requirement is greatly reduced, thus eliminating the problem of maintaining lasers running at single mode. Even partially coherent light may be used.

° It provides a wider and more controllable range senstivity, thus allowing larger deformation to be measured. Holography is too sensitive for many practical NDT measurements.

° The requirement of recording media resolution is much lower, thus allowing faster and less expensive photographic films to be used. Even vidicon may be used.

Shearography, however, is less adaptive to 3-D shapes of large depth variation.

Shearography and Holography vs conventional techniques

One major difference between these optical methods and the conventional NDT techniques is the method of revealing flaws. Techniques such as dye penetrant, magnetic particles are enhanced visual means for inspecting surface flaws; techniques such as radiography and ultrasonics reveal internal flaws by detecting material discontinuities and density inhomogeneities. Shearography and holography measure surface deformation. Holography and shearography are optical methods and the output of both techniques are fringe patterns superimposed on the object images. This provides a permanent record of the strained components. Flaws in an object create strain concentrations when subjected to stress. Both techniques detect flaws by looking for flaw-induced strain concentrations which produce anomalies in the fringe pattern. Although they measure surface deformation, both surface and internal flaws can be detected. This is because that internal defects, unless very far from the surface, also influence surface deformations. Both shearography and holography are quite effective for the detection of material imperfections such as voids, cracks, inclusions, and evaluation of adhesive joints, composites, etc. Both methods enjoy the advantages of being noncontacting, whole field, and hence high inspection rate. One major limitation of shearography and holography is the need to apply additional stress to reveal flaws.

Practical methods of stressing

Both shearography and holography is based on the comparison of two states of strains in the object. Ideally, it is desirable to impose stresses identical to the stress state found in service so that only defects located in the high stressed region will be revealed and cosmetic defects are ignored. However, exact duplication of actual loading conditions is difficult because excessive rigid body motions during stressing must be prevented. Both shearography and holography have a very limited tolerance to rigid body motion. Rigid body motion results in decorrelation of speckles which deteriorates the fringe visibility. Stress methods that would not cause excessive rigid motions and are commonly used today include: internal pressurization, thermal excitation, vibrational excitation, and vacuum. The choice depends on materials and the type of structures. For example, internal pressurization is a natural choice for pressure vessels; vacuum is ideal for soft materials such as rubber; thermal excitation is effective for revealing adhesive joints of two different materials because of the different thermal expansion coefficients, etc.

Conclusions

Each of all the existing nondestructive testing techniques possesses one or more severe limitations. Shearography and holography are no exceptions. One major limitation of both techniques is that they are not user-friendly. The output is a fringe pattern which requires skillful human interpretation. Also at present, photographic films requiring wet processing are used. The acceptance of these techniques by industries will depend upon the successful development of automated testing processes. Shearography is relatively younger than holography; its capabilities have not been fully explored. Because of its numerous advantages over holography, shearography appears to have a higher potential of being developed into a practical nondestructive inspection tool.

Acknowledgment

This investigation was supported by the National Science Foundation (Grant CEE-8219776). The support of Dr. Gifford Albright is appreciated.

References

1. Sharpe, R.S. (ed.), "Research Techniques in Nondestructive Testing, Volume 1", Academic Press, London, 1970.
2. Sharpe, R.S. (ed.), "Research Techniques in Nondestructive Testing, Volume 2", Academic Press, London, 1973.
3. Erf, R.K. (ed.), "Holographic Nondestructive Testing" Academic Press, New York, 1974.
4. Erf, R.K. (ed.), "Speckle Metrology", Academic Press, New York, 1978.
5. Caulfield, H.J. (ed.), "Handbook of Optical Holography", Academic Press, New York, 1979.
6. Vest, C.M., "Holographic Interferometry", John Wiley & Sons, New York, 1979.
7. Hung, Y.Y., "Shearography: a new optical method for strain measurement and nondestructive testing", Optical Engineering, Vol. 21, No. 3, pp 391-395, 1982.
8. Ebbeni, J. (ed.), "Industrial Applications of Holographic Nondestructive Testing", SPIE, Vol. 349, 1982.

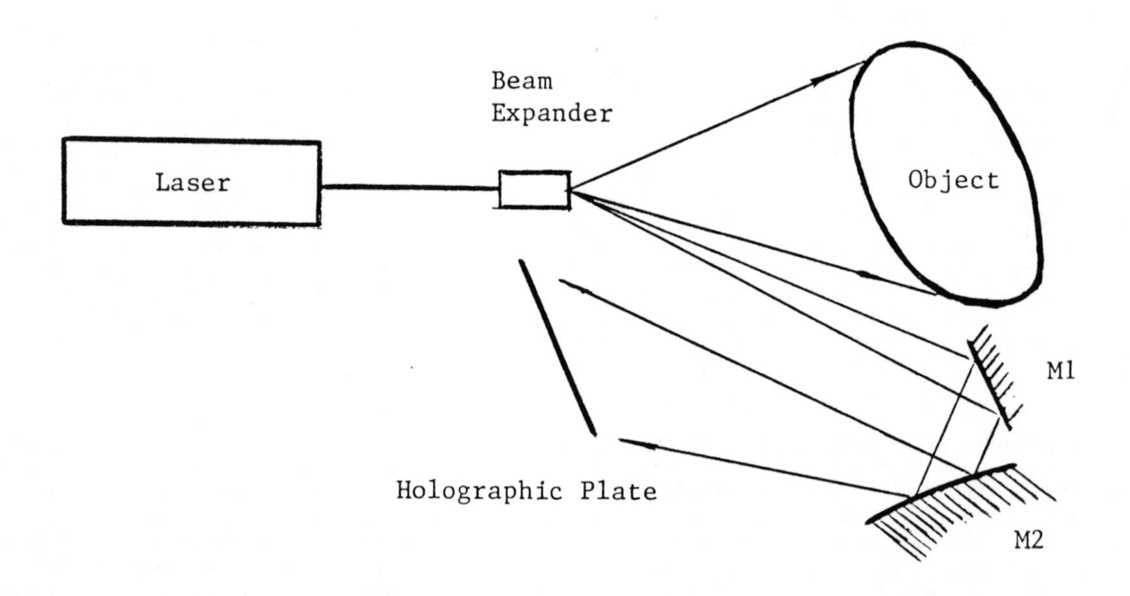

Fig. 1 Schematic of holographic recording

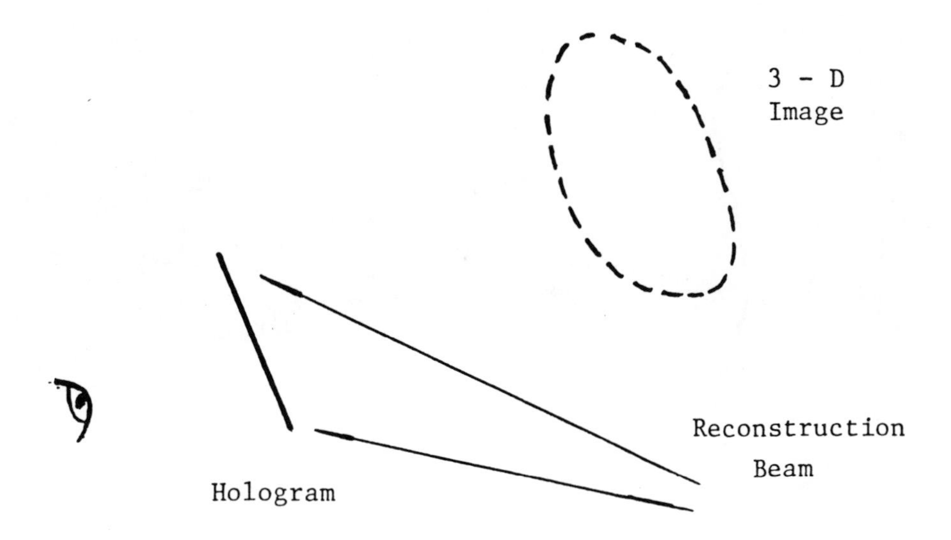

Fig. 2 Holographic reconstruction

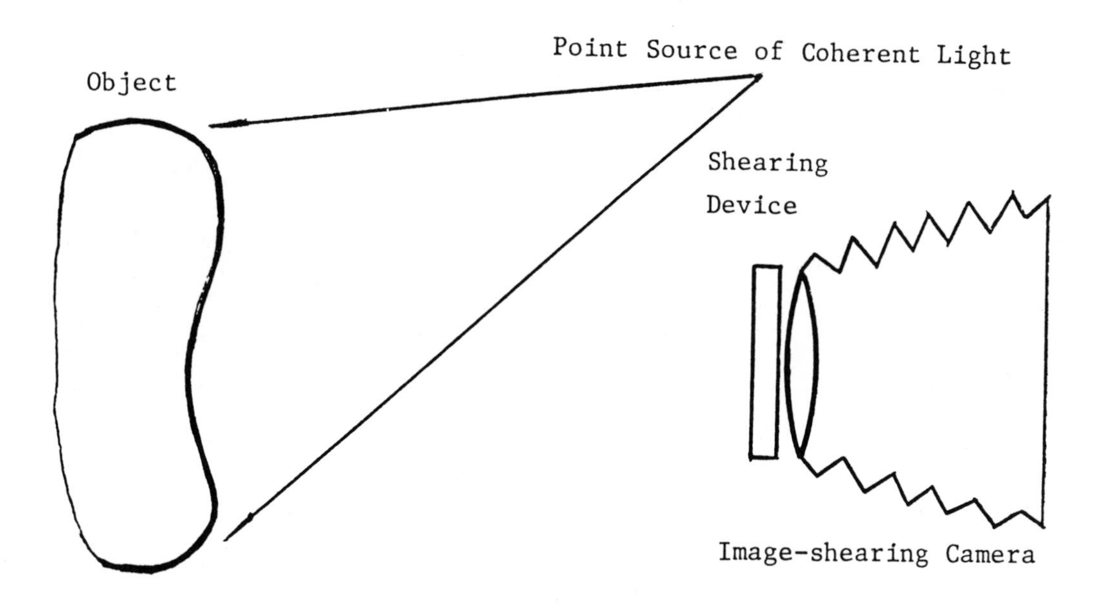

Fig. 3 Typical set-up of shearography

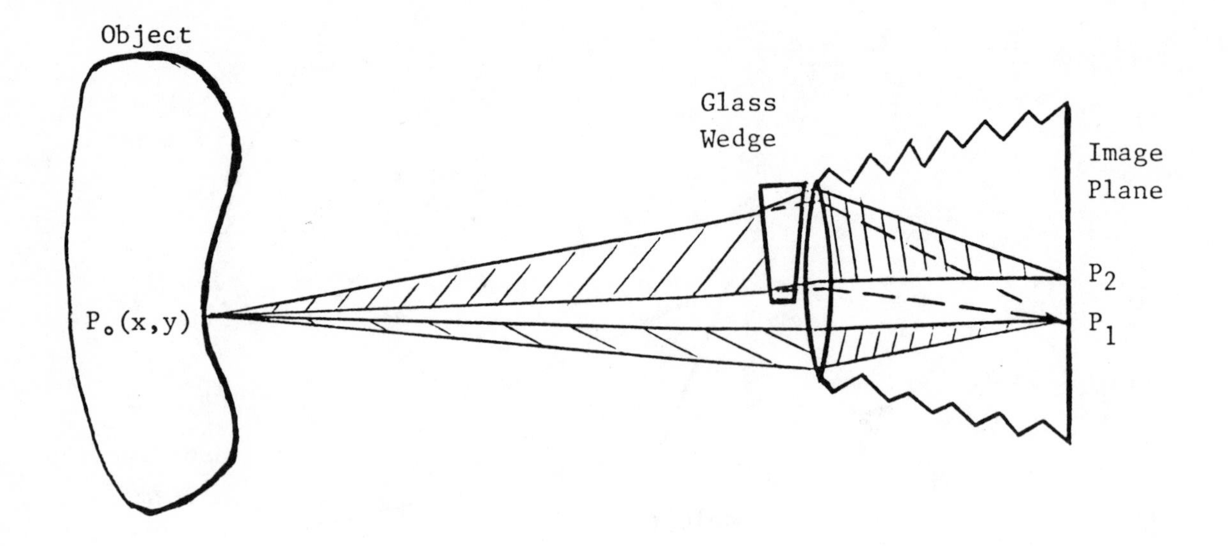

Fig.4 The image-shearing camera

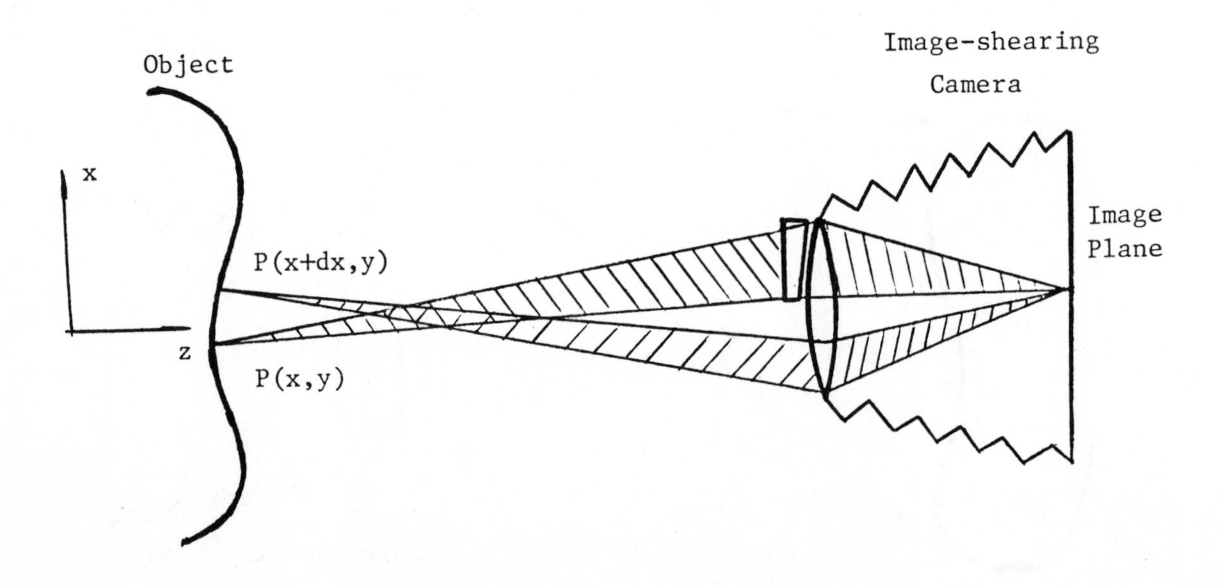

Fig. 5 Two neighboring object points are brought to meet in the image plane

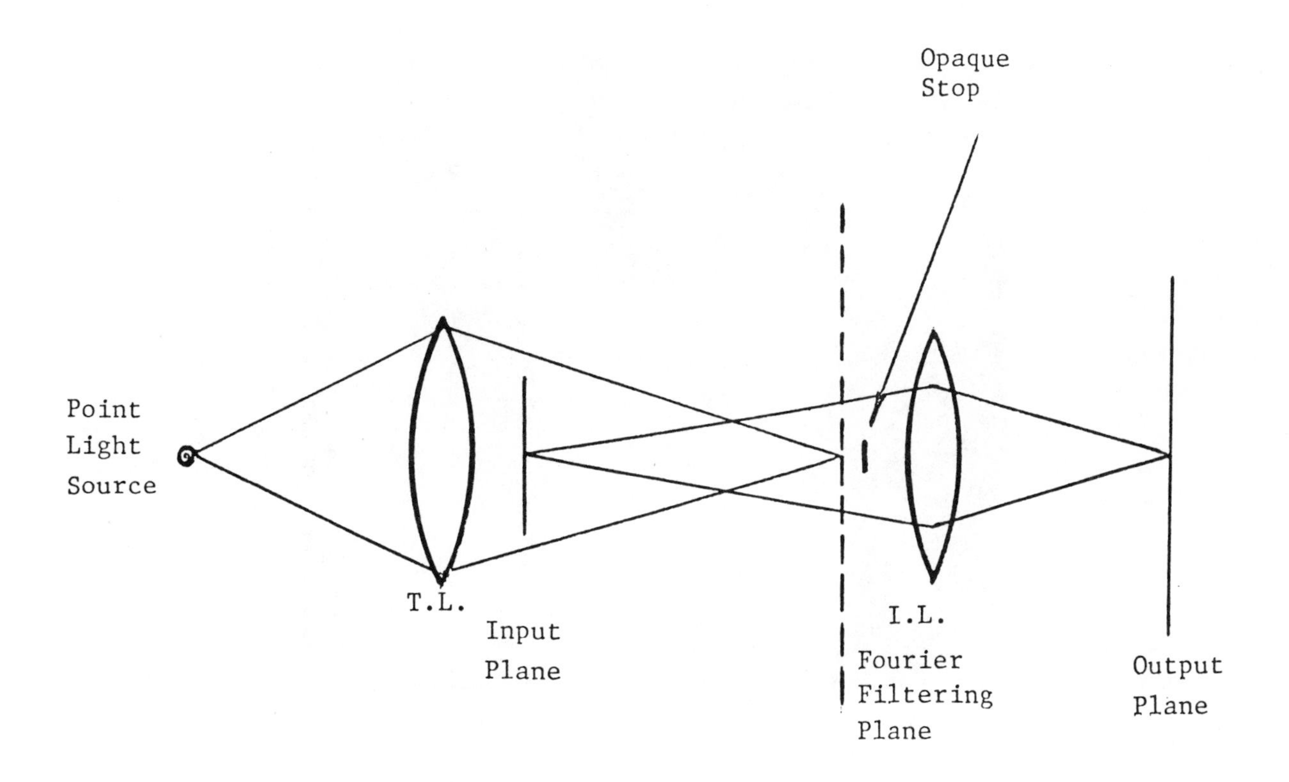

Fig. 6 The optical high-pass filtering

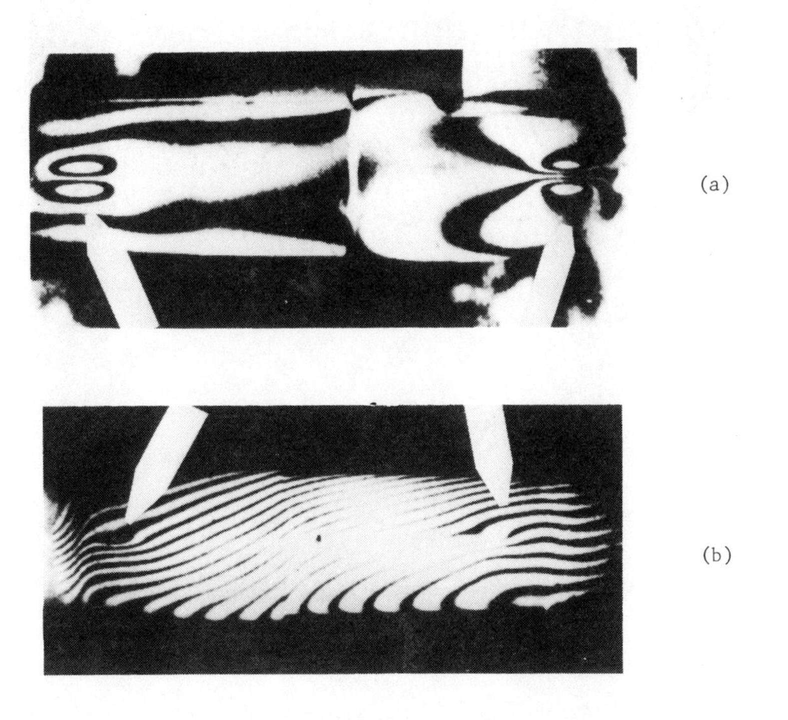

Fig. 7 Two cracks in a shell (a) shearographic fringe pattern
(b) holographic fringe pattern

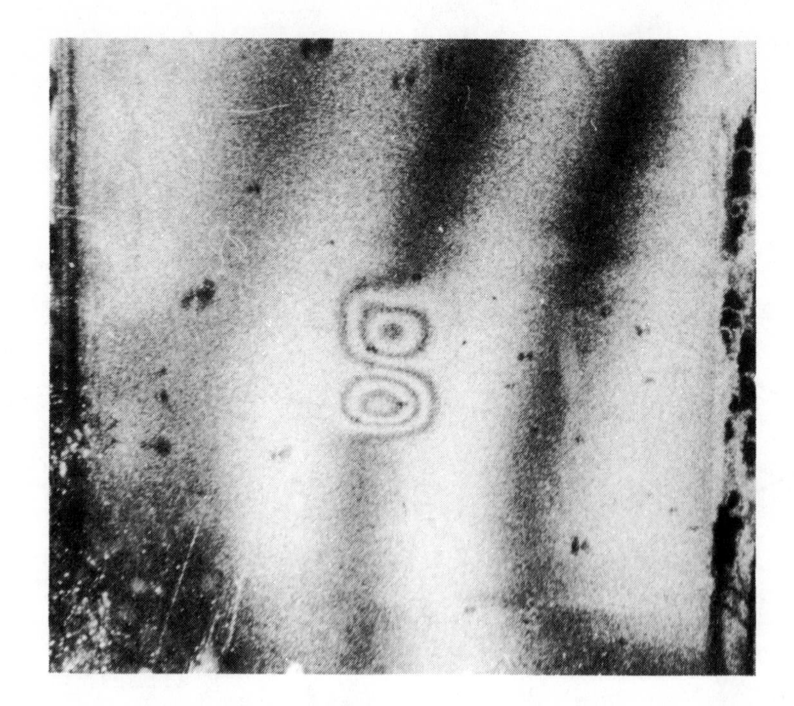

(a) shearography

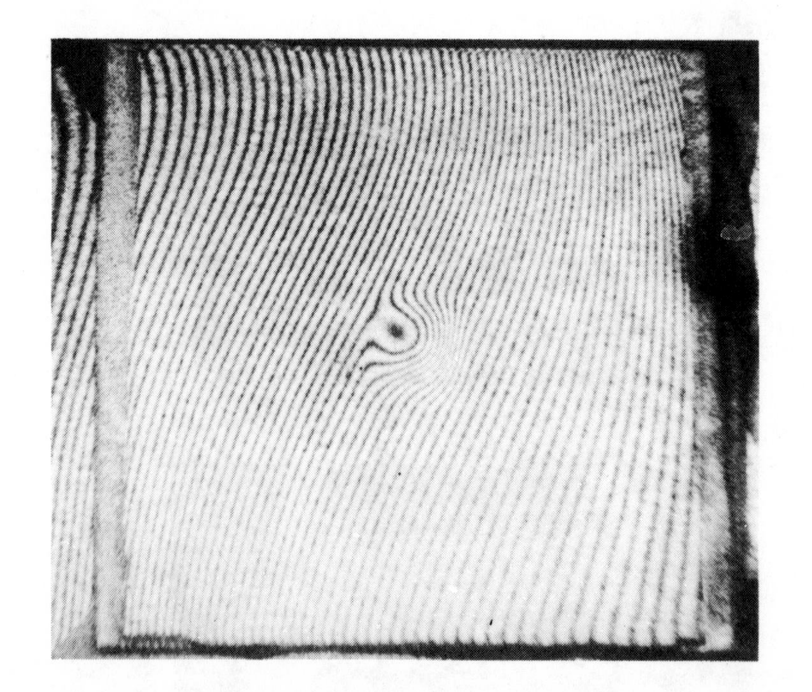

(b) holography

Fig. 8 A disbond at the interface of a metal/elastomer adhesive joint

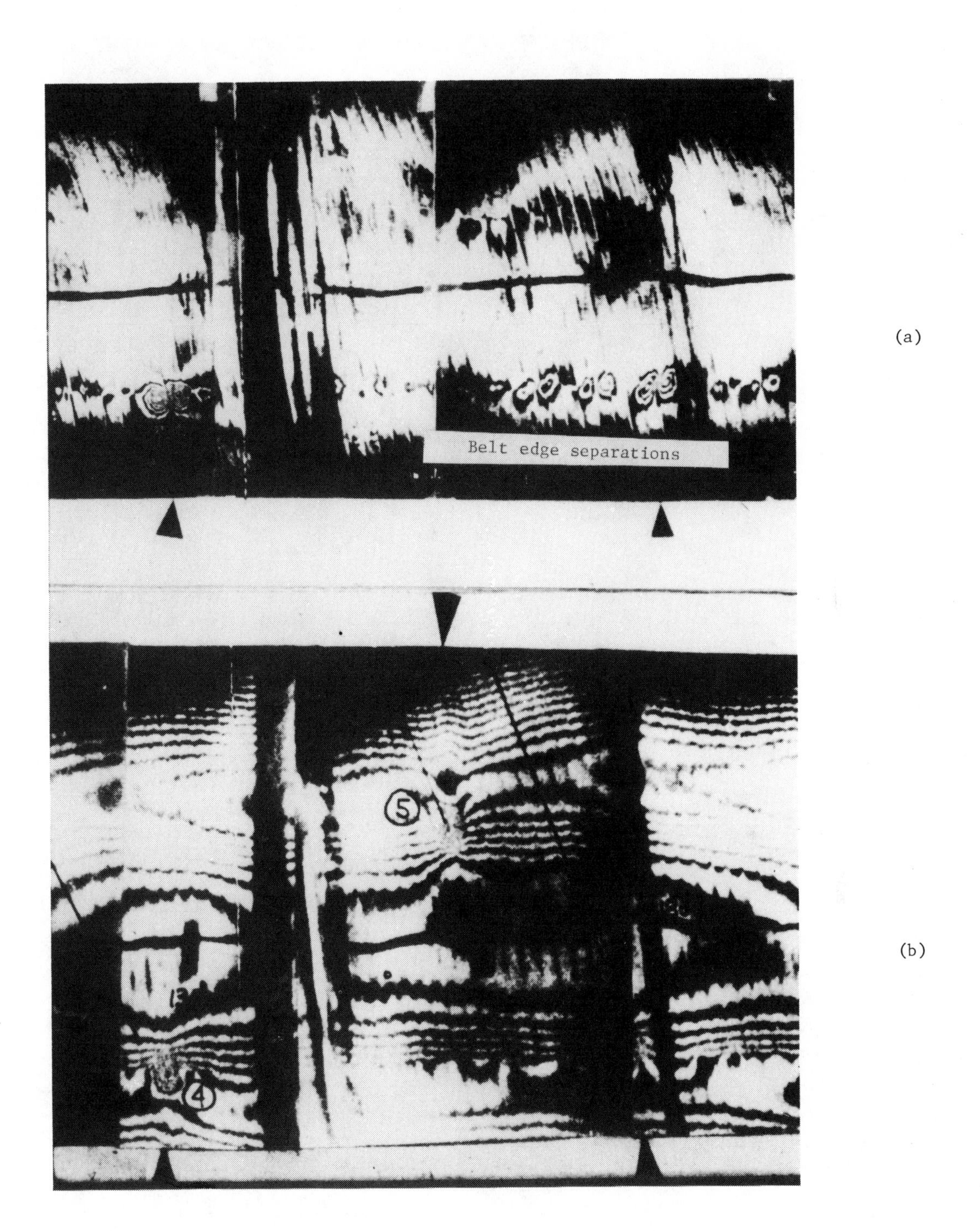

Fig. 9 Belt edge separations in a truck tire (a) shearography
(b) holography

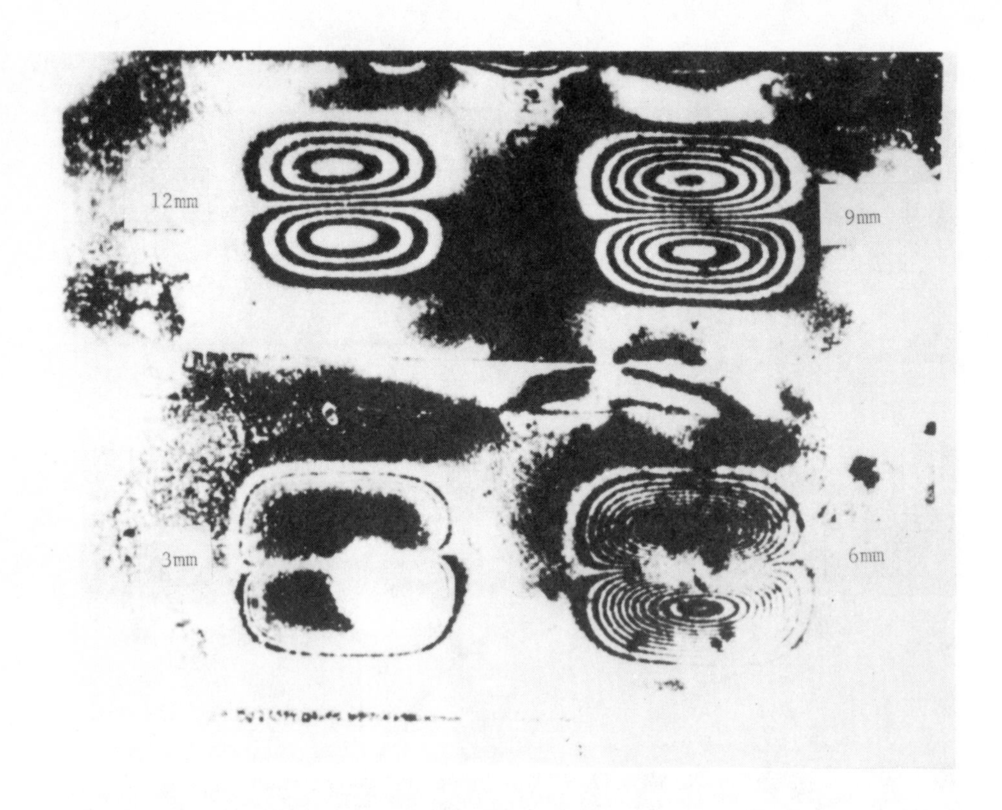

Fig. 10 Separations at the various depth

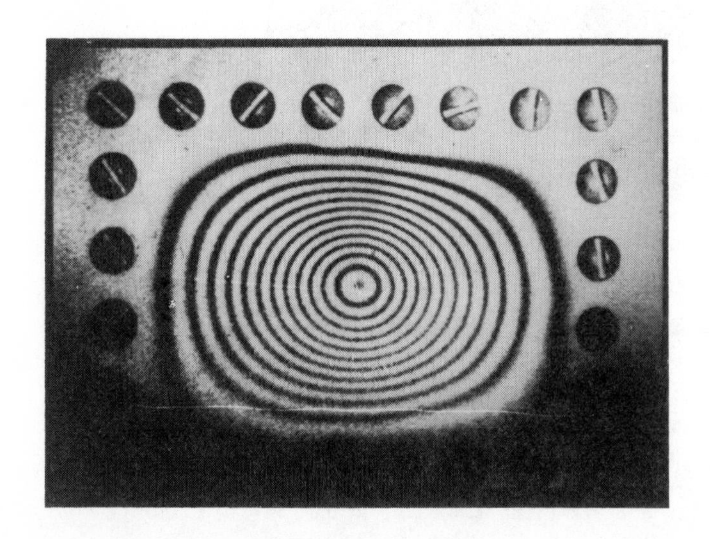

Fig. 11 Holographic fringe pattern depicting deflection of the plate

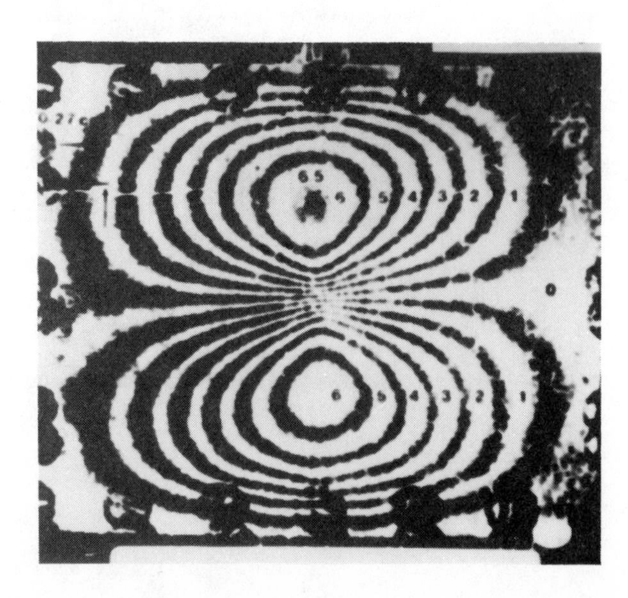

Fig. 12 Shearographic fringe pattern depicting deflection gradient

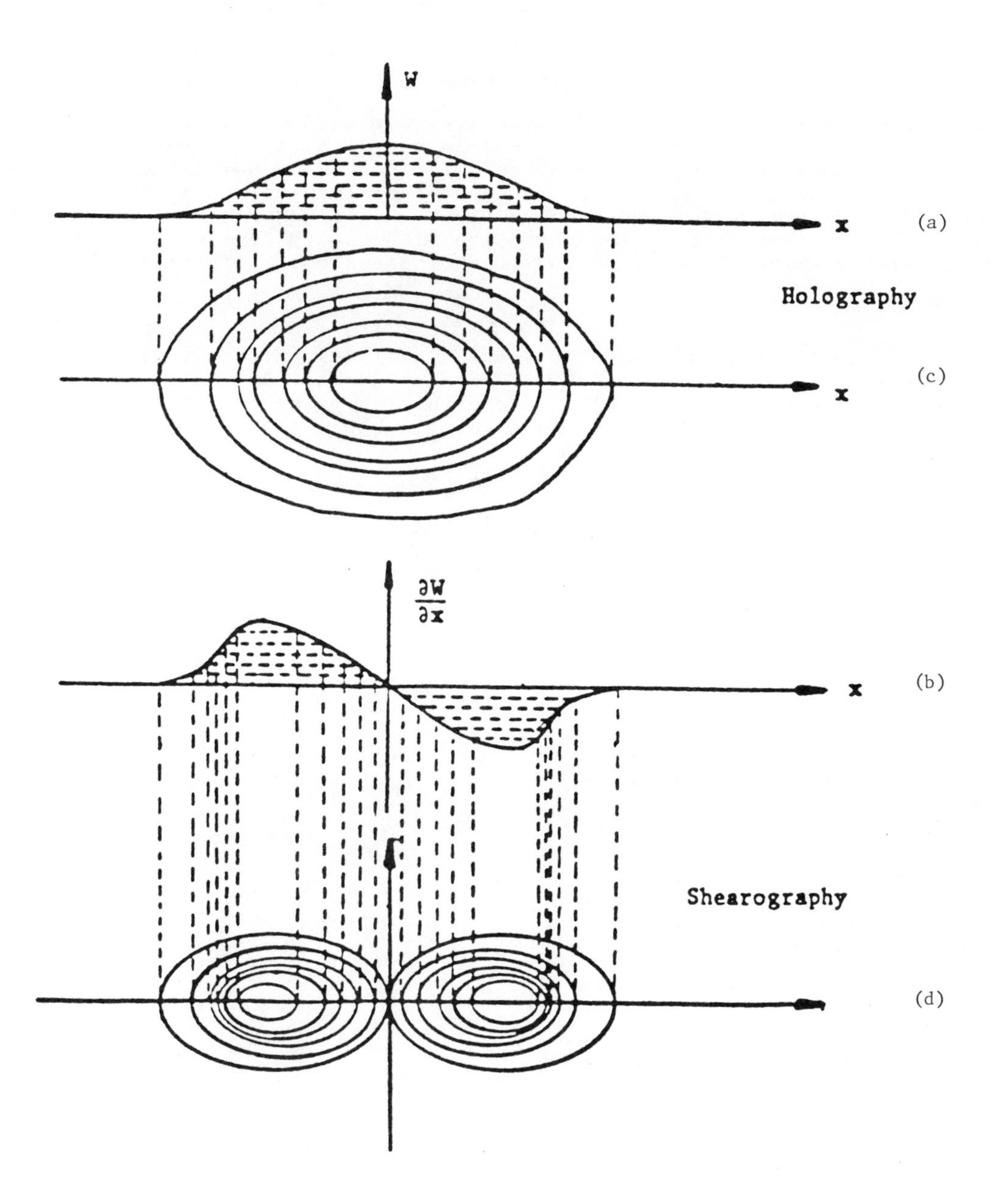

Fig. 13 Illustration of single concentric fringe pattern in holography and double concentric fringe pattern in shearography

Holographic NDT and Visual Inspection in Production Line Applications

Werner P. O. Jüptner, Th. M. Kreis

BIAS - Bremer Institut für angewandte Strahltechnik
Ermlandstr. 59, D-2820 Bremen 71, W.-Germany

Abstract

Production line applications of non-destructive testing (NDT) methods demand detailed investigations not only of the problem to be solved but also of the suitability and capability of the chosen method. For this aim a classification of the NDT methods into relative and absolute ones is presented. The results of an experimental comparison of different NDT methods applied to defect detection in glass-fiber reinforced plastics tubes are demonstrated. Two methods are given special consideration with regard to their applicability in production line: the visual inspection and the holographic interferometry.

Introduction

Holographic non-destructive testing (NDT) and Visual Inspection, that means to compare one of the most modern with the oldest NDT technique at all. But there is another important difference in the two methods: All non-destructive methods can be classified in relative and absolute ones, table 1. To explain this, a basic view to NDT is necessary.

Table 1. Non-destructive testing methods, schematically

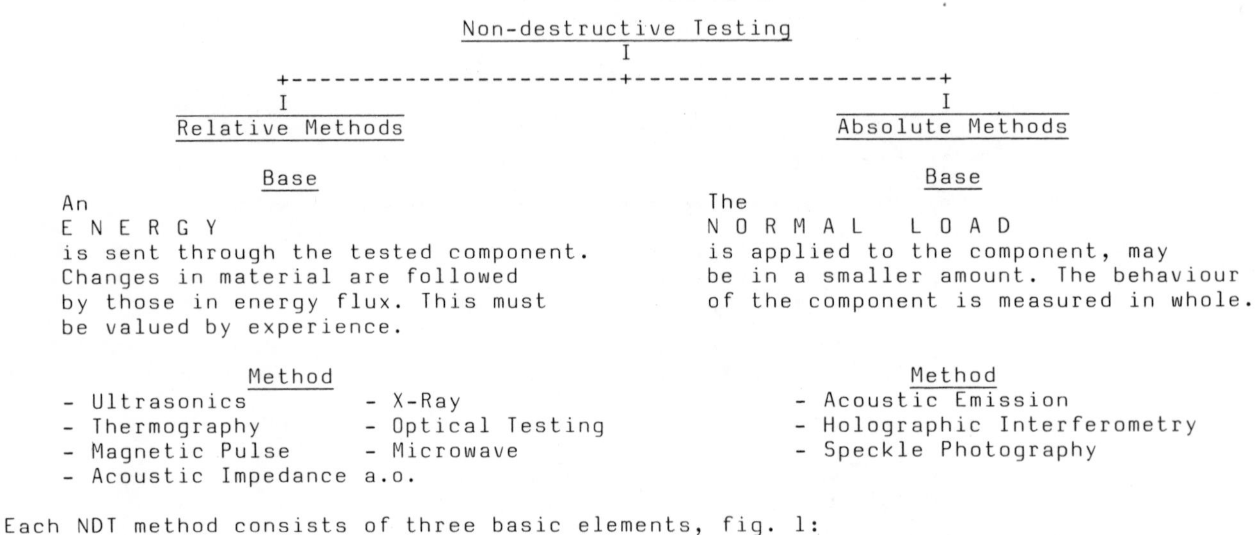

Non-destructive Testing

Relative Methods	Absolute Methods
Base	**Base**
An E N E R G Y is sent through the tested component. Changes in material are followed by those in energy flux. This must be valued by experience.	The N O R M A L L O A D is applied to the component, may be in a smaller amount. The behaviour of the component is measured in whole.
Method	**Method**
- Ultrasonics - X-Ray - Thermography - Optical Testing - Magnetic Pulse - Microwave - Acoustic Impedance a.o.	- Acoustic Emission - Holographic Interferometry - Speckle Photography

Each NDT method consists of three basic elements, fig. 1:

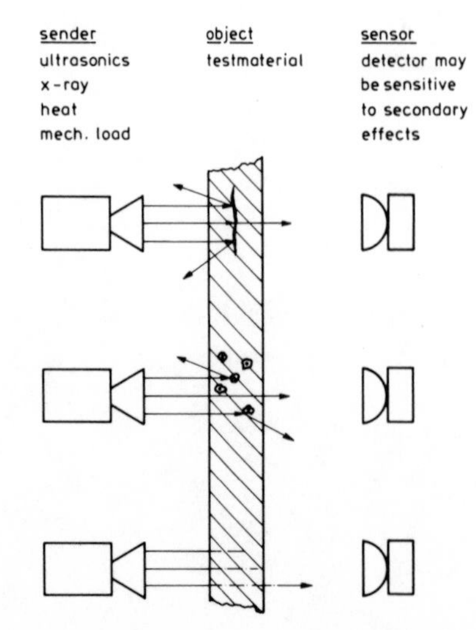

Figure 1.

Principle of nondestructive testing

- The sender (emitter) puts any energy into the test object. The energy can be in the form of ultrasonics in US-testing, X-rays in X-ray testing, heat in thermographic testing etc. In holographic NDT in most cases a mechanical load is applied, introducing deformation energy into the specimen.

- The test object transfers the energy either to another surface or back to the input surface. The transfer of the energy - the attenuation, the scattering, the transformation or else - depends on the material properties and the geometry of the specimen.

- The receiver records the transferred energy and converts it into a detectable signal.

Before starting the non-destructive testing of a given object the influence of the change of material properties on the energy transfer must be known from research and development work. If during the test a change of energy flux is observed, the tester relates it to known effects in order to find a defect. The fact is, that this detection procedure of a defect cannot classify into "good" or "bad", it only detects a change. Normally there is no relation between the test and the operational load of the component. Since most of the NDT methods only compare the detected changes of material properties relatively to a model, the methods can be classified as "relative" ones. One of these methods is the visual inspection. A collection of these NDT methods is given in table 1.

On the other hand there are testing methods, which apply the operational load to the component and detect inadmissible deformation or even crack propagation. In this case the real behaviour during the operation can be predicted. By this, it is possible to declare absolutely, that the component is "useable" or "not useable" regardless of the existence of a defined defect. Such NDT methods therefore may be classified as "absolute" ones. One of the absolute methods is the holographic NDT.

This difference between relative and absolute NDT methods should be considered in the test philosophy: By relative NDT methods one can expect to detect material changes , by absolute NDT methods one can expect to detect the operational behaviour. Before solving a new problem, all preliminaries and consequences must be checked for new. In most cases the response to the energy transfer must be evaluated especially for the test object. Furtheron the influence of detected defects on the practical behaviour should be estimated. In this case reliable results of nearly all NDT methods can be expected.

This paper reports on visual testing and holographic NDT in different applications. A comparison is presented in a special case: Visual inspection and holographic interferometry were applied beside other NDT methods to a glass-fiber reinforced plastics (GRP) tube in a cooperate research work[1].

Visual inspection

Visual inspection is the evaluation of image or optical data either detected by a human eye or more adequate for industrial application by video or line scan cameras. To determine the detectable quantities for the visual inspection a review of the interaction between light and materials is necessary[2]: If light incides to the surface of the test object, it splits into different portions, fig.2: The light is reflected, transmitted and absorbed.

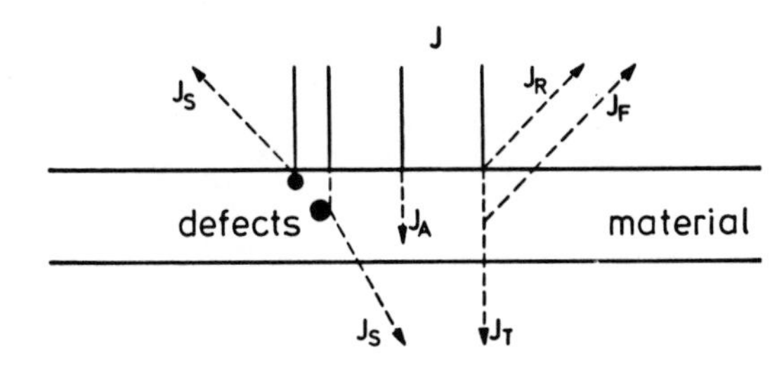

Figure 2.

Light interaction with material.

The primarily transmitted light may be scattered forward or backward; it may be absorbed and reemitted by a fluorescence effect. In visual inspection the various materials differ in the percentage of the different portions of the light: e.g. glass will transmit nearly all the light, while a metal surface will reflect or absorb it. The reflected part of the light carries information of the surface geometry and roughness, fig. 3: mirror like surfaces reflect the beam without changing the contour and the law of specular reflection is valid. Rough surfaces scatter the light around the reflection angle. The difference can be measured by using different apertures for the detection optics. Additionally, geometric defects can be localized by dynamic detection, fig. 3, righthand.

The transmitted light may be partially or totally absorbed, deflected or scattered, fig. 4. The absorption is ruled by the exponential law. The absorption coefficient depends on the material properties and the wave length of the light. A change of the absorption coefficient indicates a material change.

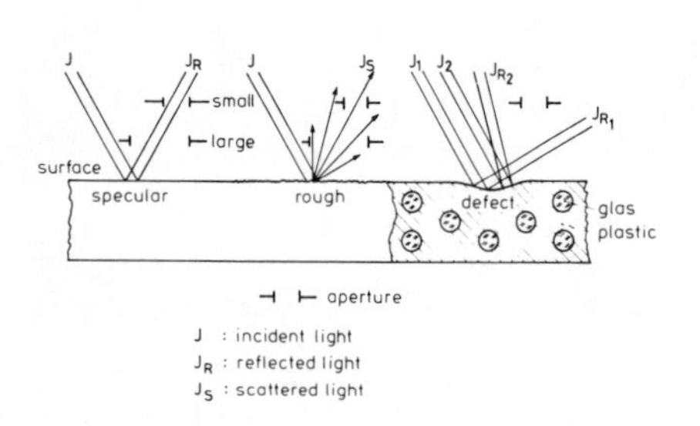

Figure 3. Reflection and scattering on a surface

Figure 4. Absorption, scattering and deflection inside material

Visual inspection of phosphoric layers on metal sheets

The test problem was to detect bad phosphoric layers in an automobil production line[3]. In order to meet industrial conditions, the specimen were tested using white light illumination and video camera observation, fig. 5. The first step was to measure the back scattered intensity over one or more lines in the video image with the result, that the surface showed stripes whenever the layer was bad and -vice versa- the layer was bad when there were stripes. The practical solution was to evaluate the gray value histogram: one peak in the histogram characterizes a good layer, two or more peaks indicate a bad one. The method was tested in production line. Disturbances by the environmental illumination could be eliminated by colour filters.

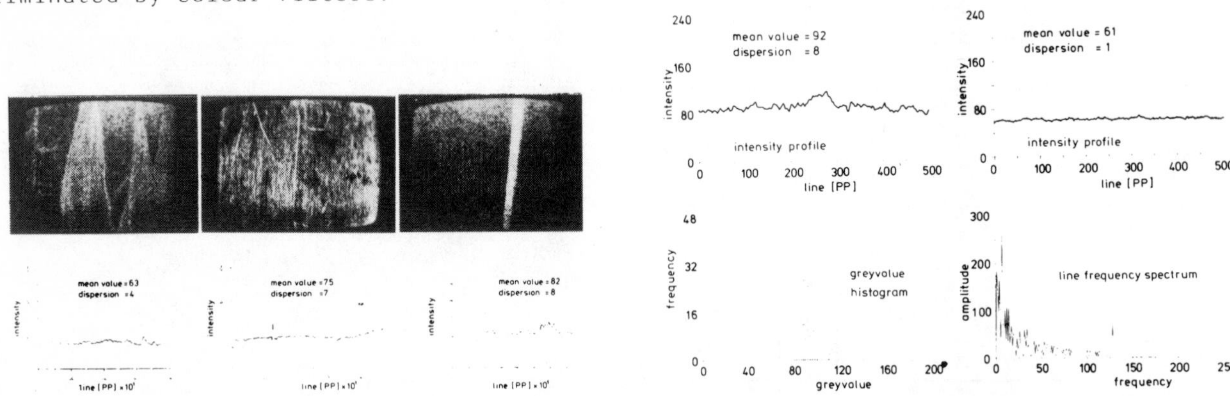

Figure 5. Video images and intensity distributions in visual testing of phosphoric layers.

Visual inspection of GRP tubes

A basic research work was done on GRP tubes, which were produced by filament winding in nine layers[1]. For this investigation several sets of GRP tubes with local defects, periodical defects or material changes were prepared. Every set of tubes had the same variation of defects. The tubes were tested with the different NDT techniques in different companies. So the state of the art of the NDT techniques could be evaluated. The result of the comparison will be given lateron.

The list of defects is given in table 2. Some defects were given in different intensities, e.g. dry cuts were prepared in the three intensities with 1, 3 and 5 layers cutted: For example, the three layers dry cut was produced by first preparing six layers, then partially hardening the tube, cutting three layers and finishing the tube[4].

Table 2. List of defects

Tube Typ	Defect Type	Defect Description
1	Reference tube	: defect free, no material change
2	Local defect	: dry cuts, internal, three intensities
3	Local defect	: fiber knots, internal, two intensities
4	Periodical defect	: missing fiber band, three intensities
5	Global defect	: dry internal layers, two intensities
6	Local defect	: impact, external, one intensity
7	Global defect	: exchange of plastic matrix
8	Global defect	: exchange of glass fibers

The optical testing was done by scanning with a laser line by line the tube and measuring the transmitted and reflected light[5]. A first test with red (He-Ne-laser), green (Ar-Ion-laser) and blue (Ar-Ion-laser) light resulted, that the red light gives the best fit for this problem, table 3. For the valuation, three quantities were measured, table 3: the change of global transmission or reflection against the reference tube, the noise of the transmission during the scanning and typical local signals.

Table 3. Results of visual testing

Tube	ΔTr	Noise	Defect Signal	Remarks
1	Reference	47 %	Tr.: Re.:	Reference tube, local defects
2	- 11 %	56 %	Tr.:	Changed, no significant defect
3	- 28 %	42 %	Tr.: = Δ Δ red: 35 % Δ green: 27 % Δ blue: 21 %	3 local defects, typ. signals
4	+ 20 %	59 %	Tr.: Re.:	3 local defects, typ. signals
5	0 %	47 %	Tr.: 130 mm 130 mm	Periodical transm. change
6	- 55 % - 84 %	120 % 200 %	Tr.: Tr.: 65 mm	Low transmission, high noise periodical and unperiodical
7	+ 20 %	47 %	Tr.:	High frequency noise

The valuation of these quantities enabled a detection of all the local or global defects or material changes. Based on these results a production line test system was proposed, which consisted of the projection of a line of white light line for illumination and a video image-analysis system for evaluation.

Holographic interferometry

An equal set of tubes was tested by holographic interferometry[6]. The load was internal gas pressure starting with a certain basic pressure and loading with a difference pressure of 0,3 MPa. The holographic set-up was a usual laboratory one, fig. 6. The typical result for the reference tube is shown in fig. 7, for a tube with three local

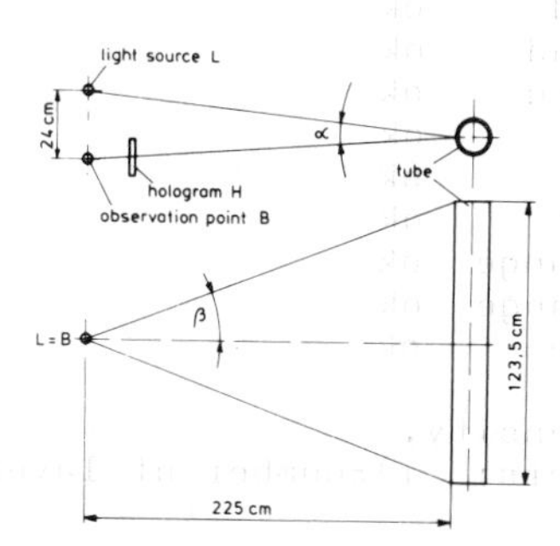

Figure 6. Holographic setup[6]

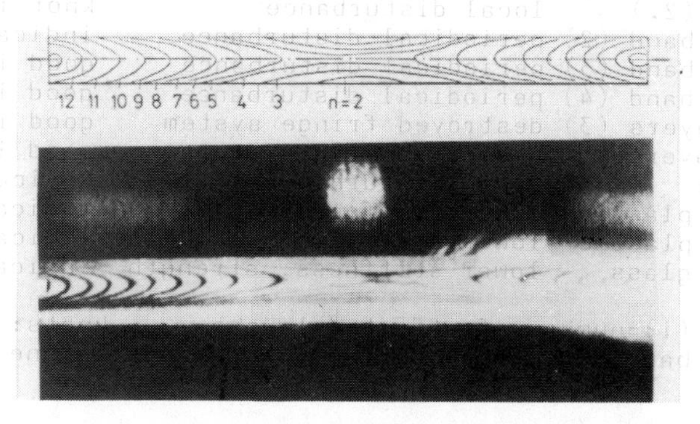

Figure 7: Fringe system, reference tube[6]

defects in fig. 8, for a tube with periodical defects in fig. 9 and for a tube with global defects in fig.10. The results of the holographic testing are summarized in table 4, which confirms a good capability for defect detection. Only in one case of material change no detection could be achieved.

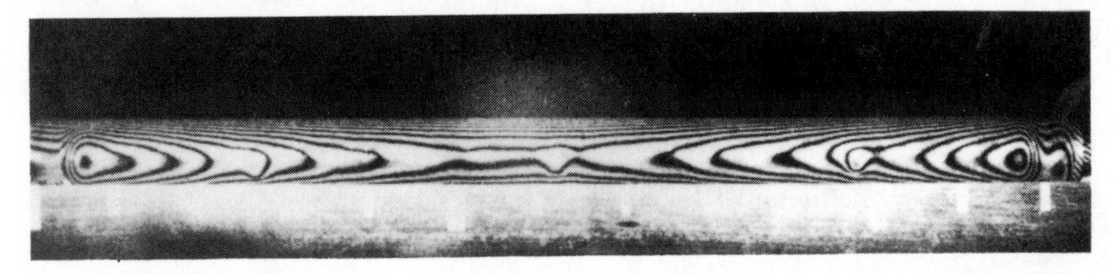

Figure 8. Holographic fringe system, GRP tube, three local defects[6].

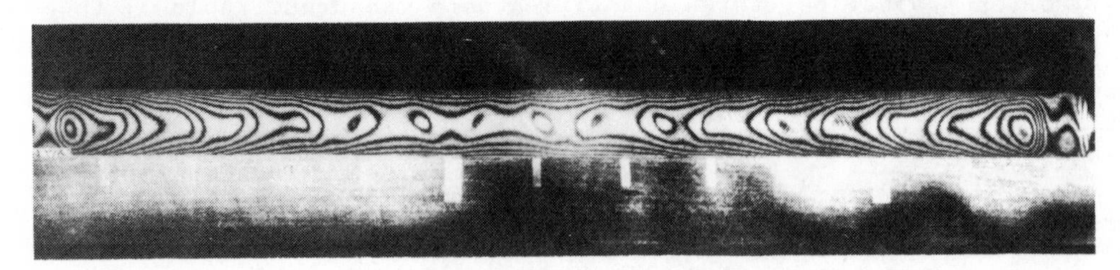

Figure 9. Holographic fringe system, GRP tube, periodical defect[6].

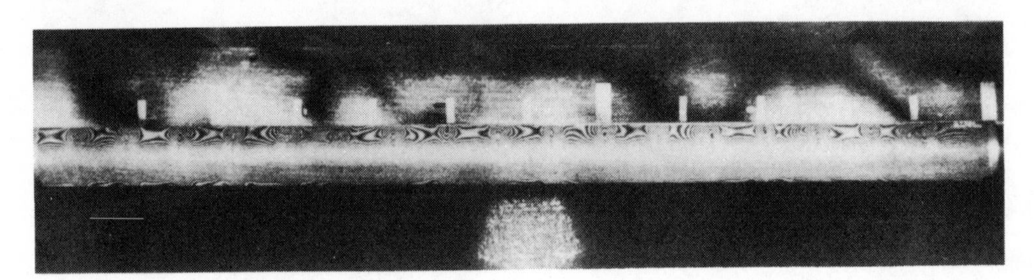

Figure 10. Holographic fringe system, GRP tube, material change[6].

Table 4. Results of Holographic NDT

Defect Type	Defect Indication	Valuation (Project Leader)	Remarks
Reference	defect free	basic fringe system	reference
Cuts (1)	local disturbance	hardly detectable	wrong, only guessed
Cuts (3)	local disturbance	cut indication	ok, needs training
Cuts (5)	local disturbance	good cut indication	ok
Knots (1.)	local disturbance	good knot indication	ok
Knots (2.)	local disturbance	knot indication	partially ok
Miss. band (2)	periodical disturbance	indication missing band	ok
Miss. band (3)	periodical disturbance	good indic. missing band	ok
Miss. band (4)	periodical disturbance	good indic. missing band	ok
Dry layers (3)	destroyed fringe system	good indication	ok
Dry layers (5)	destroyed fringe system	good indication	ok
Impact	local disturbance	indication local defect	ok
Wrong plastic	lower stiffness	indication material change	ok
Wrong plastic	lower stiffness	indication material change	ok
Wrong glass	lower stiffness, strength	Indication glass change	ok

Cuts: (i)=number of affected layers, knots: (i)=relative intensity,
miss. bands: (i)=number of missing bands in one layer, dry layers: (i)=number of layers

In production line application the holographic NDT shows the following problems:

- When the test was performed all equipments were laboratory set-ups and even today production line test machines are an exception.
- When the test was performed no automatic evaluation of fringes was available and just up today the identification of defects cannot be done automatically.
- The test is quite expensive compared, e.g. to the visual inspection.

The task of the test was the detection of defects. Taking into account that the holographic NDT has the capability to detect inadmissible deformations under operational load - it is an absolute NDT method - the task should be to valuate the deformations.

Comparison of different NDT techniques

During the research work different NDT techniques were applied to identical sets of tubes. On the base of the documented test results the defect detection was valuated by a point system with the following quantification:

0 pts: Tube is wrongly valuated, the defect is not detected.

1 pt : Changes can be recognized, detection not sure.

2 pts: Defect can be detected by trained persons, detection not sure in quality and intensity.

3 pts: Defect can be detected, detection not sure in quality and intensity.

4 pts: Defect can be detected, quantification can be done by trained persons.

5 pts: Defect can be detected and classified without restriction.

The results are summarized in table 5. Two facts are remarkable with regard to the sum of points: The result of the same NDT technique can differ between "useful" tube and "unuseable" tube, e.g. in US or Visual Inspection. This depends on the good or bad adaption of the method to the problem. The other fact is the bad result of Acoustic Emission Analysis (AEA). Simplified the AEA works as follows: The operational load is applied to the object. If the defect initiates a crack propagation, noise can be detected and indicates an "unuseable" object. Therefore it is an absolute NDT technique, which directly enables the valuation: an uncritical defect will not be detected.

Table 5. Comparison of NDT Results

Defect Type	X-Ray	US		Holgraphy		Thermogr.		AEA	Optics	
		1	2	1	2	1	2		1	2
Reference	5	5	5	5	5	5	5	5	5	5
Cuts (1)	5	0	5	0	0	4	0	0	1	1
Cuts (3)	5	1	5	3	4	5	4	2	3	4
Cuts (5)	5	1	5	5	5	5	5	5	4	5
Knots (1.)	5	4	5	5	5	5	5	3	5	5
Knots (2.)	5	4	5	3	3	5	5	3	5	5
Miss. band (2)	5	4	5	5	5	5	1	2	5	5
Miss. band (3)	5	4	5	5	5	5	3	0	5	5
Miss. band (4)	5	4	5	5	5	5	3	2	4	5
Dry layers (3)	4	5	5	5	4	5	5	3	4	5
Dry layers (5)	4	5	5	5	3	5	5	5	4	5
Impact	5	4	5	5	5	5	5	3	5	5
Wrong plastic	0	4	4	4	5	4	0	3	0	5
Wrong plastic	4	2	5	4	0	5	4	0	5	5
Wrong glass	5	4	5	5	3	5	5	4	5	5
Sum of points	67	51	74	64	57	73	55	40	56	70

Future Aspects

The result of an NDT test must be the valuation of the defect in regard to the criticality. The holographic interferometry enables this valuation. Recent results in automatic evaluation of fringe systems and the present research work will arise the capability to measure directly the stresses and stress intensities. In this way, fracture mechanics can be applied to NDT. With the introduction of fracture mechanics a production line non-destructive valuation of components will be done.

Acknowledgement

The investigations were sponsored by the German Ministry of Defense. The authors wish to thank all companies, which took part in this research work.

References

1. Jüptner, W., Stadler, H.-J., Kleberger, W.A., Investigations in Non-Destructive Testing of GRP Tubes and Project Management of the Experimental Studies, Report Nr. T/RF52/RF520/42016 (German)
2. Kellner, R., Jüptner W., Sepold, G., Eine neuartige optische Prüfmethode für glasfaserverstärkte Kunststoffe, DGaO, Berchtesgaden 1978
3. Jüptner, W., Automatisierte Prüfung von lackierten Oberflächen, Tagung "Lackierroboter", Böblingen 1982
4. Stadler, H.-J., Preparation of GRP Tubes with Defined Defects, Private communication
5. Kellner, R., Untersuchungen zur optischen zerstörungsfreien Prüfung von Rohren aus glasfaserverstärktem Kunststoff, Bericht Nr. T/RF52/RF520/42016/17
6. Steinbichler, H., Prüfung von GFK-Hochdruckrohren mittels Holografie, Bericht Nr. T/RF52/RF520/42016/03

Holographic and nonholographic NDT for nuclear and coal-fired power plants

David L. Mader

Ontario Hydro, Research Division
800 Kipling Ave., Toronto, Canada M8Z 5S4

Abstract

The use of holographic interferometry for nondestructive testing (NDT) in nuclear power plants and coal plants is discussed in terms of test code requirements, and is compared with conventional NDT techniques. Holography provides a useful laboratory tool to support the electric utility industry through measurement of deformation, movement, expansion, and vibration. Although optical holography may not have sufficient signal to noise ratio in the power plant environment for the detection of defects buried in thick walled pressure vessels or pipes, it offers a means to measure slight deformations so that pressure vessel integrity could be evaluated directly through response to pressure.

Introduction

Mechanical failure in power plant equipment may result in forced outages, costly repairs and lost production, and could cause personal injuries. Such failures often arise from the growth of flaws which originate from small defect sites. The objective of nondestructive testing (NDT) is to detect significant defects before they cause failures. This review considers the use of holographic interferometry for NDT in nuclear power plants, with an emphasis on pipes since they are a basic and widely used type of component. As exemplified by Fig. 1, flaws on the inside surface of a pressure component can be detected.

The impetus for development of holographic interferometry for NDT lies in its noncontact nature and its coverage over the full field of view with one hologram. By contrast radiography covers a field of view equal to the film size, and ultrasonics would miss any flaws which may happen to lie between probed locations.

Development of holography has progressed to the stage where laboratory measurements and observations can produce useful results. Field work requires special procedures and has been done in a limited number of cases.

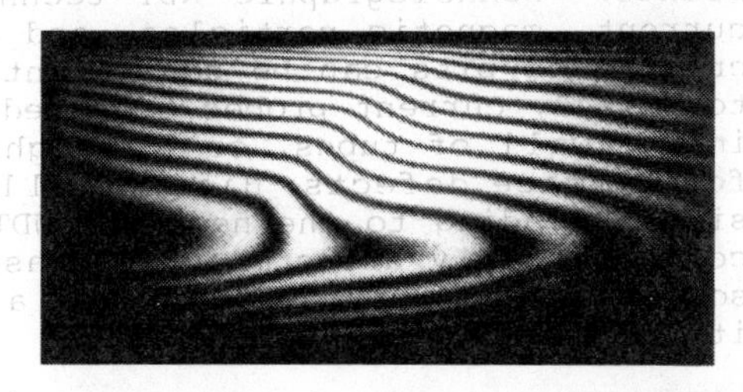

Fig. 1. Kink in the fringe pattern is due to spiral fabrication weld on inside wall.

While the author has no references to the actual detection of a defect in a nuclear power plant using holographic interferometry, several useful laboratory experiments have been done. In a project on the repositioning of certain spacers around pressure tubes in a Canadian heavy water nuclear reactor, there was a need to determine whether or not these tubes were liable to be damaged by magnetic pulsing. A holography experiment was able to prove that pressure tube deformation, if any, would be less than one micrometer. In a companion project on the relocation of spacers using vibration to move them, real-time holographic interferometry was able to verify that the exciters were producing the desired vibration mode. In a classic vibration visualization experiment on a power turbine blade of a type that was experiencing field failures, vibration modes with large amplitudes were found in the area of cracking.

On a question of damage to piping during maintenance when sections of water filled pipes are isolated from the rest of the system by freezing a plug of ice in them, both holography and strain gages were used. The strain gages, being limited in number, gave spot readings of strain during the entire freeze/thaw cycle. On the other hand, holography gave the deformation over the entire field of view, but only after the entire cycle was over, since the fringe pattern was first disturbed by the cooling and then obliterated by the frost. Both techniques were able to provide evidence that damage to the pipes in question was unlikely.

Strain measurement with pressure loading has been done by Mader[1] using math model fitting in which a simulated fringe pattern is fitted to the observed data. Then the parameters in the model constitute measured values of the actual physical conditions, such as an average strain value. The method accommodates rigid body motion by including it in the model. In the same work, thermal expansion coefficients were obtained for a sample of extruded zirconium nuclear reactor pressure tubing. As expected, the axial expansion coefficient was distinct from the radial one, due to extrusion.

Hsu[2] wrote on an experimental study of the ability of holographic interferometry to obtain the material properties of nuclear fuel cladding tubes at elevated temperature. He found, for example, that for the same number of deformation fringes, the pressure required at 650°C was 0.2% of that needed at 600°C.

Defect detection is a valuable potential application of holography. An experiment on a section of boiler tubing from a coal-fired generating station has demonstrated the ability of holography to detect areas of erosion or corrosion. However, a similar experiment failed to detect known subsurface hairline cracks, as discussed later.

A field use capability would add immeasurably to the attractiveness of holographic interferometry. Since interferometry responds to changes in the optical path in the two arms of the interferometer, including changes in the index of refraction of the intervening air as well as surface displacement of the object due to stress or rigid body motion, there are several considerations involved in obtaining measurements. The optical path difference must be stable to within half of a wavelength during the time required for exposure. Heat waves in the air need to be controlled. Rigid body motion must be controlled or compensated for. Present day equipment for field use consists of special double-pulse lasers, and suitable shutters and film transporters. Each individual pulse is short enough to freeze any motion. The second pulse is emitted before any excessive motion can occur. What is captured, then, by such a double exposure hologram is a sample of rigid body motion or of a vibration pattern, the sample period being the time between the pulses. To extend the technique to NDT, Vest,[3] for example, has suggested that impulse loads could be applied, and the laser pulses could be triggered when the strain wave reaches the defect location.

Regulatory agencies specify NDT techniques to be used in periodic inspections of generating stations operated by electric utility companies. For example, the American Society of Mechanical Engineers (ASME) Nondestructive Testing Code for Pressurized Components may be used in whole or in part, with Section XI being used for inservice inspection of nuclear plants.[4] Nonholographic NDT techniques routinely used are ultrasonics, radiography, eddy current, magnetic particles, and dye penetrants. Where the surface is accessible, surface cracks and pits can be conveniently detected by application of inexpensive visual indicators. Eddy current probes are used for the same purpose in inaccessible regions such as the inside wall of tubes, or for tightly closed cracks. These techniques have high sensitivity for surface defects. Historically it has been found that welds are liable to be defect sites, leading to the need for NDT on welds. Buried defects in welds or other locations are conventionally detected by ultrasonic waves, or by radiography using X-rays or radioactive sources. Acoustical holography, a phase sensitive form of ultrasonics, is starting to find its niche.

Optical holographic interferometry provides a means to observe the change in the exterior shape of an object when it is stressed. Significant subsurface defects would be manifest through their effect at the surface. Thus, optical holography could detect defects provided these have a greater effect on the observations than noise and systematic errors.

This report puts emphasis on testing requirements to guide thinking for any proposed new test method. Nondestructive testing is a live field with ongoing development in both holographic and nonholographic techniques.

Components to be tested and test code requirements

A power plant could be subdivided into steam raising equipment, rotating machines, electrical equipment, and the balance of the system. Concerns with the rotating machines (steam turbines and electrical generators) include dynamic balancing, stress corrosion cracking, and deterioration of insulation. The steam raising and handling equipment is subjected to water and steam at elevated temperature and pressure, and to deposits of crud which may cause accumulation of corrosive chemicals. In coal-fired plants, the water filled tubes in the boiler suffer erosion from the flame and fly ash. While all of these areas may provide opportunities for new NDT techniques, this review will consider only the inspection of the pressure boundary of the steam raising components, with emphasis on pipes since they are both widely used and are relatively simple to analyze. Testing requirements are concentrated on welds, since these are the most probable failure sites in pressurized components. Cracks are a major type of defect which must be detected and monitored.

Cracks in pipes are generally oriented either circumferentially (hoop direction) or axially (longitudinal direction) as seen in Fig. 2. Since the circumferential stress is twice as great as the axial stress the most probable direction for cracks to grow is axial. Crack growth in the circumferential direction is favored, however, in circumferential welds joining a pipe to another pipe or other component.

Considering the maximum allowable crack size, Copeland and Riccardella,[5] for example, reach two conclusions which may be paraphrased as follows for the case they examined:

(i) Flaws of depth less than 2% of pipe wall thickness will not grow to significant size during the life of the plant.
(ii) For a flaw of initial depth 10% of wall thickness, the crack will not grow to a critical size for well over ten years thus allowing a ten year inspection interval.

The ASME[4] Code on Nondestructive Testing of Pressurized Components, Section XI, Components in Nuclear Power Plants, considers several types of components and specifies testing techniques and maximum allowable defect sizes. All pressure retaining components are to be checked visually for leakage when the are inspected. In addition, all welds are to be examined with a suitable NDT technique. This applies to pressure vessels and to pipes.

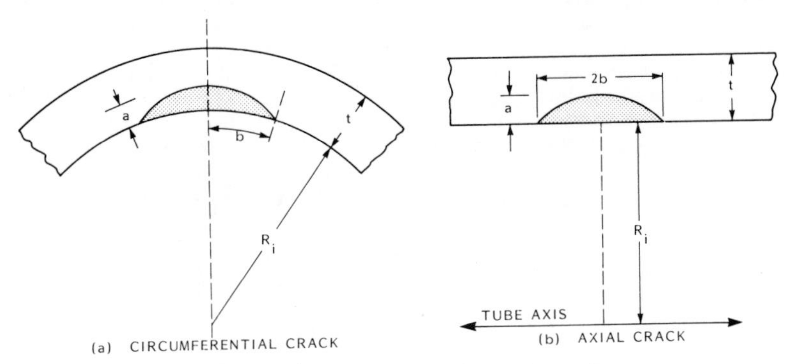

Fig. 2. Crack orientations in pipes.

Flat cracks, or planar flaws, are described by the ASME in three categories: surface, subsurface, and multiple.[4] It is assumed that the cracks have no thickness, leaving two dimensions to characterize them: **l** = 2**b**, their length, and **a**. For the surface breaking case, **a** is the width, whereas it is the semi-width for subsurface flaws. Their depth from the surface, **S**, is used to decide whether to classify a subsurface flaw as surface or subsurface. Since natural cracks have irregular shapes, rules are given in the figures below to determine the values of **l**, **a**, and **S** to use to enter tables which give allowable flaw sizes.

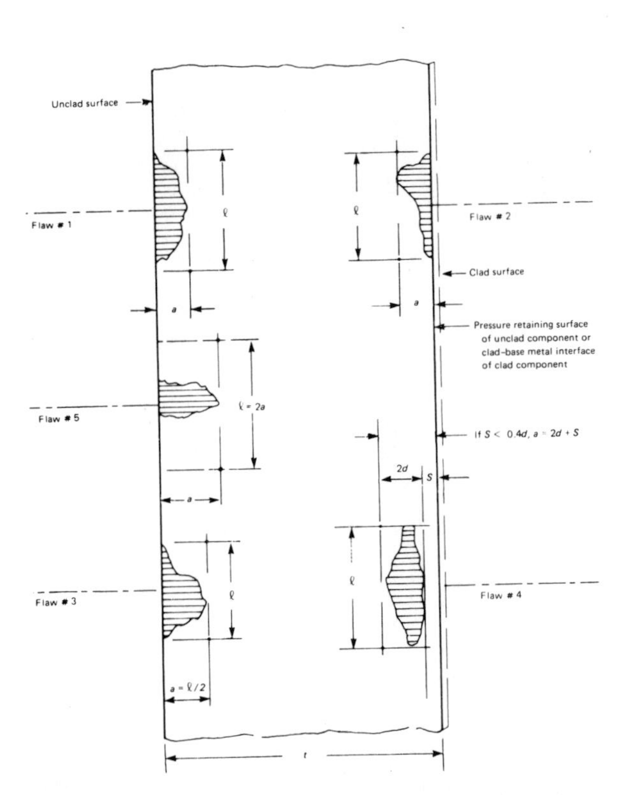

Fig. 3. Surface planar flaws, in wall of pressure vessel or pipe of wall thickness t, oriented in plane normal to pressure retaining surface. Source: ASME Fig. IWA-3310-1. Used by permission.

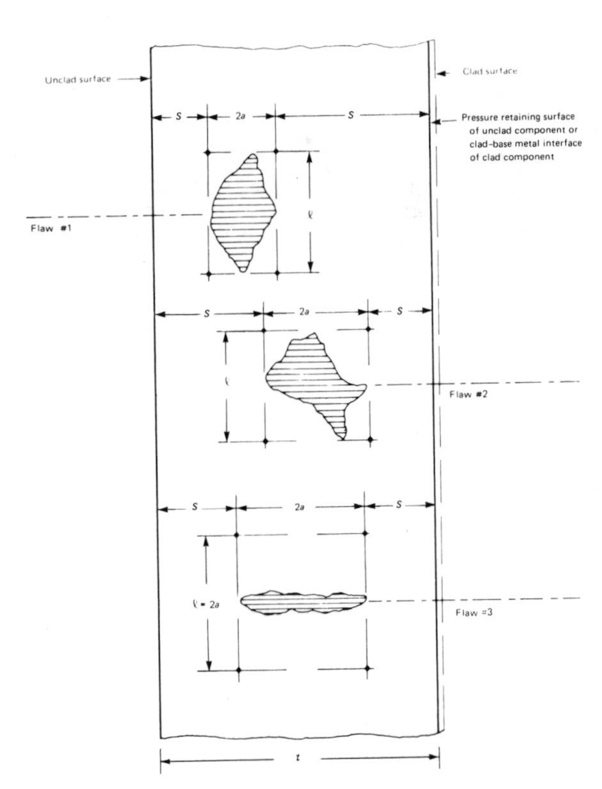

Fig. 4. Subsurface planar flaws, where **S** is greater than 0.4 **a**, oriented in plane normal to pressure retaining surface. Source: ASME Fig. IWA-3320-1. Used by permission.

Figure 3 illustrates flaw configurations and determination of dimensions **a** and **l**. Cracks on the outside unclad surface could be detected by surface detection means such as magnetic particles or dye penetrants, though volumetric inspection means such as radiography or ultrasonics would be used to determine crack depth. As a note of explanation on cladding, pressure vessels may be coated on the inside with a layer of stainless steel applied by welding. As indicated by Flaw #2, cracks in the base metal may not extend through the cladding and so may not be accessible to surface detection means. Cracks shown previously in Fig. 2 would be idealizations of a single surface breaking flaw.

Subsurface cracks are shown in Fig. 4, with a rule based assessment of their severity for different shapes. For the same area, flaws like Flaw #3 are more severe than Flaw #1 because they intersect more lines of force.

The case of multiple flaws is shown in Fig. 5, in which rules are given for combining small nearby flaws into a large single flaw for the purpose of entering the table on allowable planar indications. One reason for combining, say, X-ray indications is that the X-ray image may be incomplete with gaps left between indications even when the flaw is continuous.

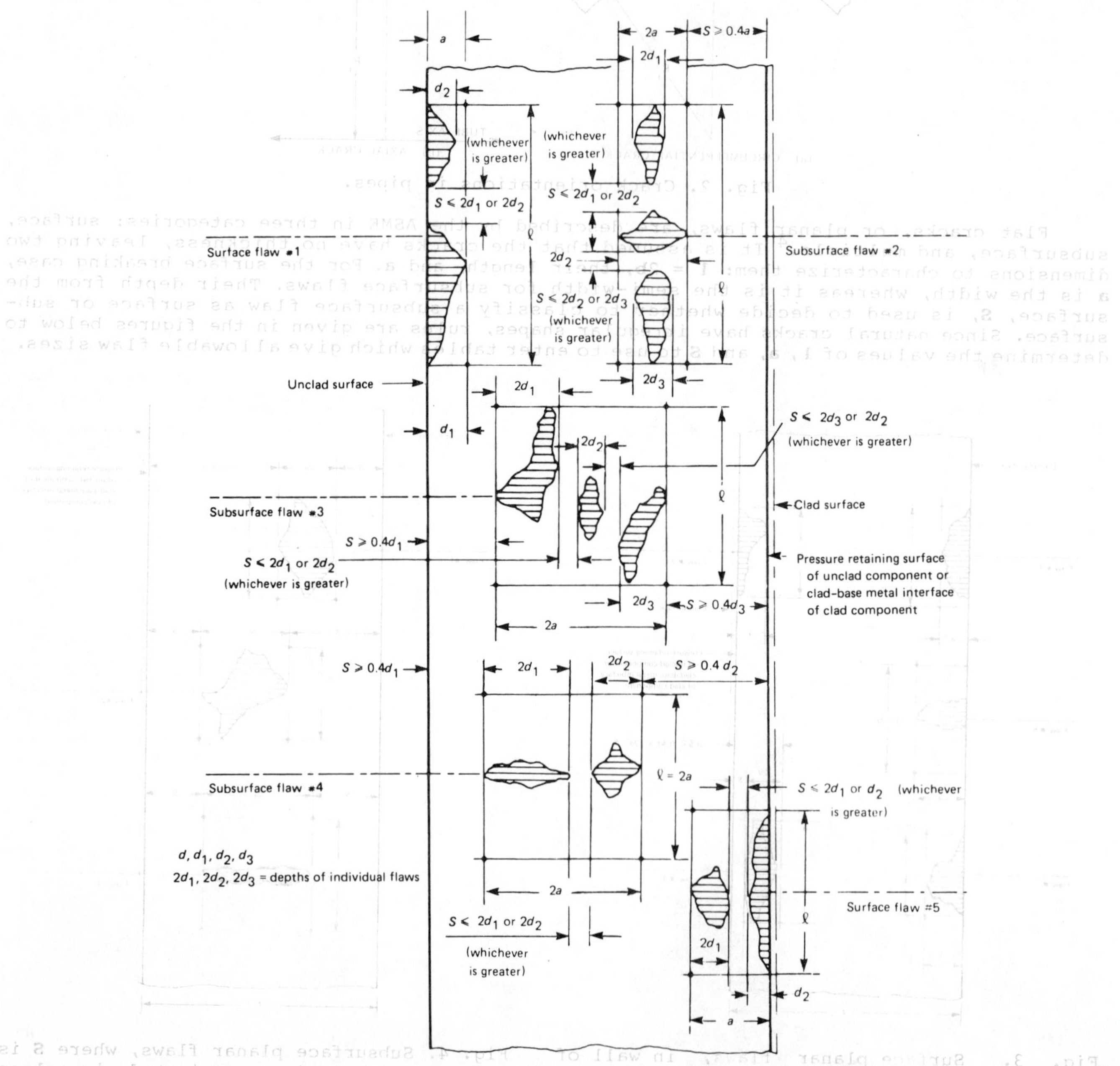

Fig. 5. Multiple planar flaws oriented in plane normal to pressure retaining surface. Source: ASME Fig. IWA-3330-1. Used by permission.

After the NDT indications have been characterized in terms of **a**, **l**, and **S**, using the rules given in the above figures, Table I is consulted (for "Class 1 Components, Examination Category B-J") to determine if the flaw is allowable, or if the pressure vessel or pipe must be repaired. Clearly any usable NDT technique must be able to detect flaws at least as small as the smallest allowable case. The smallest allowable indication seen in the table is for the preservice examination of a vessel with a 3.0 inch wall thickness with a flaw aspect ratio of 0.00 and Y = 0.4. Here, the semiwidth is 3.04%. This would correspond to a flaw of type #1 seen on Fig. 4 with **l** much greater than **a** and with the distance to the nearest wall **S** = 0.4 **a**. Any such flaw, then, with **a** over 3.04% of wall thickness would be cause for rejection of the component. The largest flaw, largest as a fraction of wall thickness, seen anywhere on the table would have a semi-width **a** = 12.5% of wall thickness.

Table I. Allowable planar indications.

Material: Austenitic steels that meet the requirements for the specified minimum yield strength of 35 ksi or less at 100°F

	Volumetric Examination Method, Nominal Wall Thickness,[1,2] t, in.								Surface Examination Method	
	0.312		1.0		2.0		3.0			
Aspect Ratio,[1] a/ℓ	Surface Indication, a/t, %	Subsurface Indication[3,4] a/t, %	Surface Indication, a/t, %	Subsurface Indication[3,4] a/t, %	Surface Indication, a/t, %	Subsurface Indication[3,4] a/t, %	Surface Indication, a/t, %	Subsurface Indication[3,4] a/t, %	Nom. Wall Thickness,[1,2] t, in.	Indication Length, ℓ, in.
Preservice Examination										
0.00	9.4	9.4Y	8.5	8.5Y	8.0	8.0Y	7.6	7.6Y	0.312 or less	1/8
0.05	9.6	9.6Y	8.6	8.6Y	8.2	8.2Y	7.7	7.7Y		
0.10	9.8	9.8Y	8.8	8.8Y	8.3	8.3Y	7.8	7.8Y	1.0	3/16
0.15	9.9	9.9Y	8.9	8.9Y	8.4	8.4Y	7.9	7.9Y		
0.20	10.0	10.0Y	9.1	9.1Y	8.6	8.6Y	8.1	8.1Y	2.0	1/4
0.25	10.0	10.0Y	9.2	9.2Y	8.7	8.7Y	8.2	8.2Y		
0.30	10.0	10.0Y	9.4	9.4Y	8.9	8.9Y	8.3	8.3Y	3.0 and over	1/4
0.35	10.0	10.0Y	9.5	9.5Y	9.0	9.0Y	8.5	8.5Y		
0.40	10.0	10.0Y	9.7	9.7Y	9.1	9.1Y	8.6	8.6Y		
0.45	10.0	10.0Y	9.8	9.8Y	9.3	9.3Y	8.7	8.7Y		
0.50	10.0	10.0Y	10.0	10.0Y	9.4	9.4Y	8.9	8.9Y		
Inservice Examination										
0.00	11.7	11.7Y	10.6	10.6Y	10.0	10.0Y	9.5	9.5Y	0.312 or less	0.2
0.05	12.0	12.0Y	10.7	10.7Y	10.2	10.2Y	9.6	9.6Y		
0.10	12.2	12.2Y	11.0	11.0Y	10.4	10.4Y	9.7	9.7Y	1.0	0.25
0.15	12.4	12.4Y	11.1	11.1Y	10.5	10.5Y	9.9	9.9Y		
0.20	12.5	12.5Y	11.4	11.4Y	10.7	10.7Y	10.1	10.1Y	2.0	0.45
0.25	12.5	12.5Y	11.5	11.5Y	10.9	10.9Y	10.2	10.2Y		
0.30	12.5	12.5Y	11.7	11.7Y	11.1	11.1Y	10.4	10.4Y	3.0 and over	0.65
0.35	12.5	12.5Y	11.9	11.9Y	11.2	11.2Y	10.6	10.6Y		
0.40	12.5	12.5Y	12.1	12.1Y	11.4	11.4Y	10.7	10.7Y		
0.45	12.5	12.5Y	12.2	12.2Y	11.6	11.6Y	10.9	10.9Y		
0.50	12.5	12.5Y	12.5	12.5Y	11.7	11.7Y	11.1	11.1Y		

NOTES:
(1) For intermediate flaw aspect ratios a/ℓ and thickness t, linear interpolation is permissible. Refer to IWA-3200(b) and (c).
(2) t is nominal wall thickness of actual wall thickness as determined by UT examination.
(3) The total depth of a subsurface indication is $2a$.
(4) $Y = (S/t)/(a/t) = S/a$. If $Y < 0.4$, the flaw indication is classified as a surface indication. If $Y > 1.0$, use $Y = 1.0$.

Source: ASME Table IWB-3514-2. Used by permission.

Thus any proposed NDT technique must be capable of at least detecting the above sizes of cracks to be useful in showing that a component meets ASME allowable requirements. In the next section, published detection capabilities of optical holographic interferometry are reviewed.

Literature survey on holographic NDT for nuclear power plants

A number of studies have been reported in the literature on laboratory simulations of defect detection in power plant components. It is to be understood that for such components holographic NDT is in its infancy and that the principle itself is at stake, so that detection of a defect in a weld, a pipe, a pressure vessel or any other component could be taken as assurance that the principle is sound.

The use of holography for weld defect detection has been studied by Katzir et al,[6] for example, who fabricated a pressure vessel with a known defect in a girth weld. They reported that the defect was not visible in the raw interferogram, but could be identified, when compared with an unflawed region, in a graph of computed displacement across the region of the defect. They report that " the difference however is quite small." They then compare computed derivatives for the flawed and unflawed cases and find greater differences.

In a study of the ability of holography to detect flaws in pipes, Martin[7] created artificial flaws by cutting small slots part way into the inside wall of a tube sample and obtained the interferogram of Fig. 6 which shows from one to three extra fringes depending on the depth of the slot.

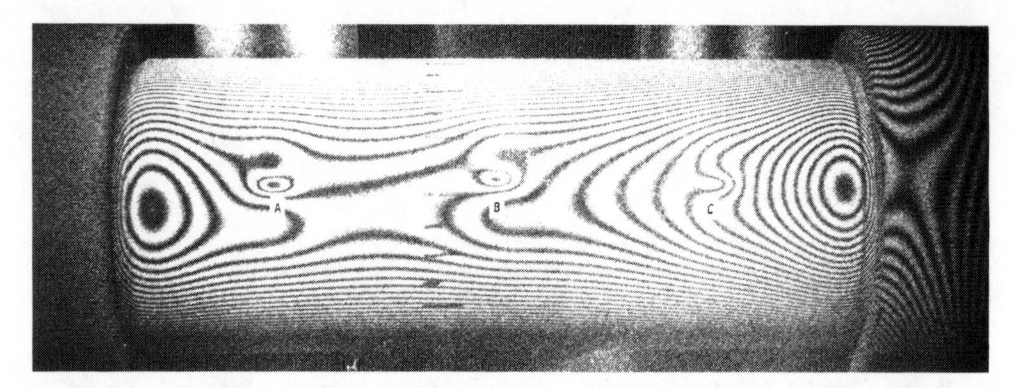

Fig. 6. Holographic interferogram obtained by pressurization of tube with three small slots on the inside wall. The slot sizes are indicated on the next figure. Source: Previously unpublished photo for 1000 psi, top view, kindly supplied by D.J.V. Martin.

Of particular value was his analysis of defect detection limits, shown in Fig. 7, in which he shows the minimum length of slot which can be detected, as a function of how deeply the slot was cut into the wall. As expected, shallow slots have to be much longer than deep ones to be detectable. For a 101 mm diameter tube with a 6.35 mm wall thickness, Martin finds that the required length rises very steeply for slot depths less than 12% of wall thickness, in effect showing that the minimum detectable flaw size (radial dimension) was about 12% in his case. His detection criterion appears to be one fringe.

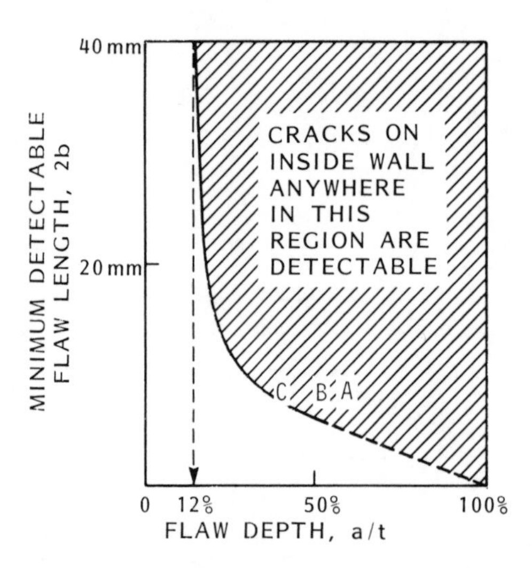

Fig. 7. Detectability of cracks on inside wall of tube. Adapted from: Martin.

Wachutka et al[8] have studied the ability of holography to detect flaws buried in the wall of a pressure vessel. Their artificial flaws consisted of either a round hole or a slot machined through a bar of steel, to simulate either an infinitely long void or crack, respectively. The bar was subjected to tension as seen in Fig. 8 (a) to simulate loads on the wall of a pressure vessel. When the bar was observed on a flaw-free side, holographic interferograms showed the displacements seen in (b). For the case of a single flaw located midway through the wall, their experimental results were in good agreement with calculations made using the finite element method (FEM).

It can be seen from the sensitivity curve, Fig. 8 (c), that for one fringe the defect semi-width **a** would be 10% of wall thickness for a round hole and 17% for a crack. For both types of flaw, surface deformation was found to be proportional to the square of the flaw size.

Turning to the ASME[4] code for cracks, the minimum allowable detection sensitivity may be estimated by considering the maximum allowable defect sizes. Orienting the X-Z plane of Fig. 8 (a) in the plane of Fig. 4 and considering the two-dimensional nature of the case studied by Wachutka et al, the length **l** would be taken as infinite so that the aspect ratio to use in Table I would be 0.00. For a flaw on the centerline as studied here, take Y = 1.0. Then the maximum allowable flaw would have semiwidth **a** of 12.5% of wall thickness, requiring detection of 0.5 of a fringe using a square law. For the smallest allowable planar indication of 7.6% for a flaw on the centerline, the detection capability would have to be at least 0.2 of a fringe. Such signals, such as 0.2 fringe, could be detected reliably if the random and speckle noise are less than, say, 0.1 fringe and if the complexity of the background fringe pattern does not obscure them.

This level of performance may be difficult to achieve under field conditions. A thorough study of environmental noise effects would be in order to ensure that holographic equipment and test conditions would be satisfactory.

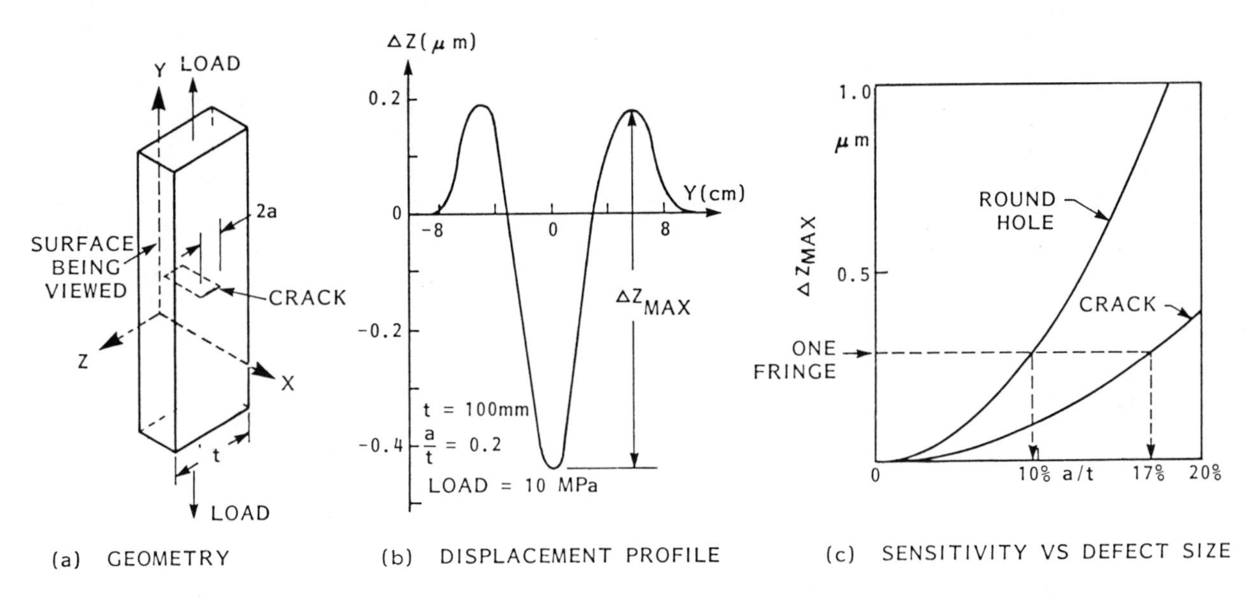

Fig. 8. Surface deformation for cracks and holes located midway through the wall. Deformation of the surface indicated in (a) is shown in (b) for the designated conditions. The magnitude of the surface effect is seen in (c) as a quadratic function of defect size. Adapted from: Wachutka et al.

Doty and Hildebrand[9] have studied the detection capability of holography on an artificial defect that they machined into the inside wall of a nuclear plant valve. They drilled a flat bottomed hole of diameter 1.11 cm into the 1.27 cm thick wall of the valve casing from the inside, and, took interferograms for each of several increments of depth. The interferogram for the last increment, when the hole was 90% of the way through the wall is shown in Fig. 9.

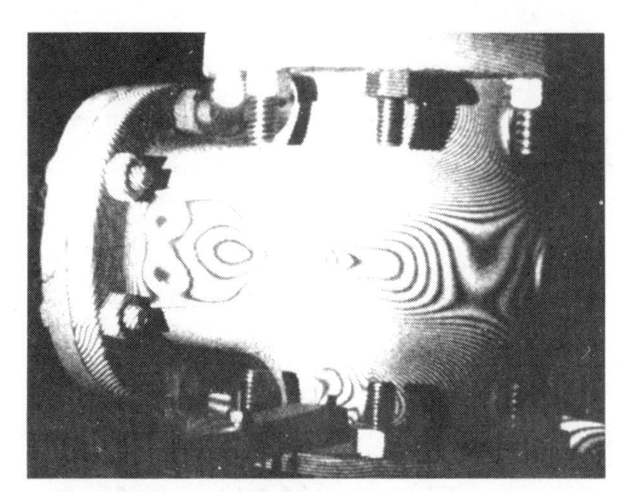

(a) Unflawed valve

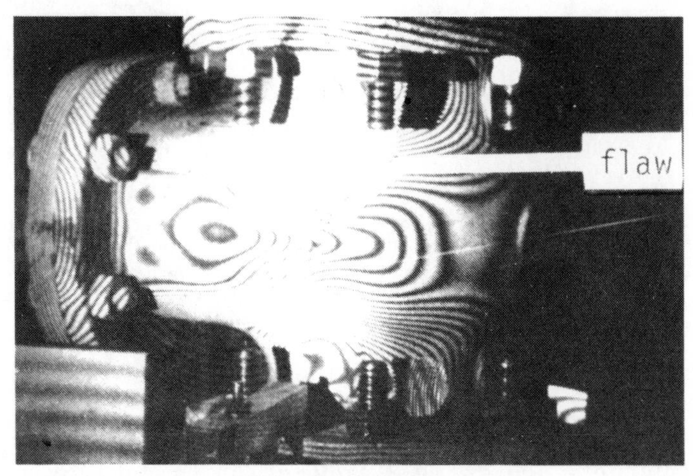

(b) Flawed valve

Fig. 9. Nuclear plant valve with void on inside wall. Interferogram for 2.8 MPa (400 psi) pressure increment. Source: Photos kindly supplied by B.P. Hildebrand.

A complicating factor in the detection of flaws by means of an interferogram such as that seen in Fig. 9 is its complexity. Even an unflawed valve, which has a complex shape, yields a complex interferogram with a number of features that attract the eye and could lead to false alarms. The flaw could be detected in the interferogram seen above when its location was known, or by comparing the interferogram of the flawed valve with one taken under the same conditions before the hole had been made.

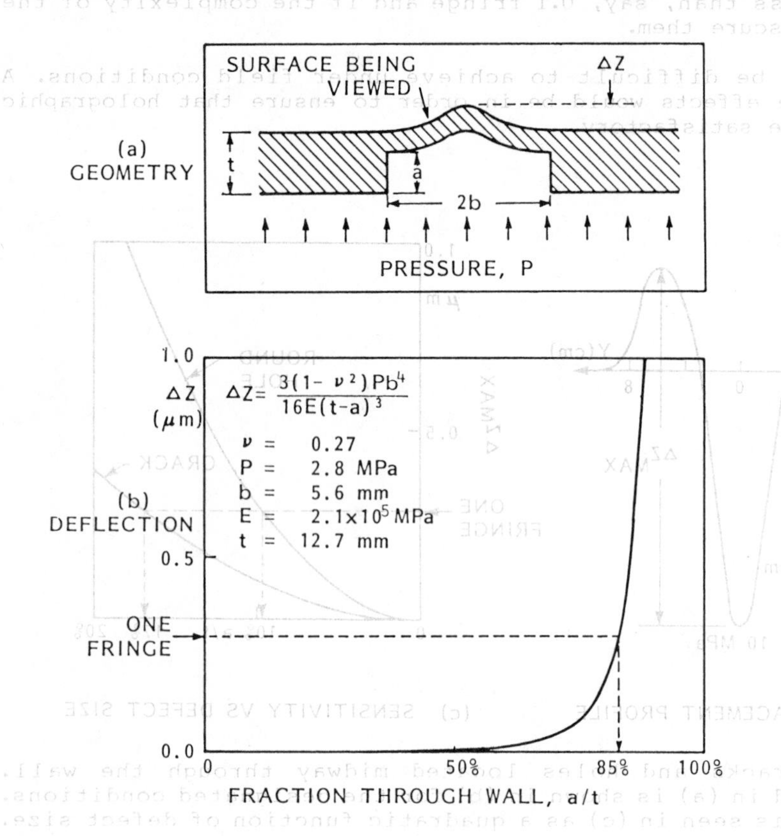

Fig. 10. Deformation due to pitting in valve body. Adapted from: Doty and Hildebrand.

According to the analysis of Doty and Hildebrand[9] shown in Fig. 10, the exterior wall deflection due to the hole would produce one extra fringe at a hole depth of 85% of wall thickness for their particular set of experimental conditions. Their formula, taken from Roark and Young,[10] for the bowing of the diaphragm formed by the remaining wall shows a deflection proportional to the fourth power of the hole diameter, and inversely proportional to the third power of the remaining wall thickness. Thus, from this formula we could calculate that to have seen the effect of the hole at a depth of 10% of wall thickness, for example, would have required detection of a change in the normal fringe pattern corresponding to 0.0046 of a fringe, or a phase change of 1.7 degree. From the experience of the author (Mader), it would require stringent control of vibration and air currents to provide reliable detection of such small phase effects. By contrast, neither X-rays nor ultrasonics would be subject to disturbance by air currents or slight vibration.

From the fourth power dependence seen above on the flaw width it could be inferred that holography has much greater sensitivity to broad areas of wall thinning than to narrow defects. Hence, applications for holography are more likely to arise in detection of broad areas of erosion or corrosion than in detection of pitting.

Literature survey on comparison of NDT testing techniques

Boyer[11] has produced a four hundred page volume on nondestructive inspection and quality control with chapters on inspection techniques using optical holography, acoustic holography, radiography, neutron radiography, ultrasonics, acoustic emission, eddy current, electromagnetic sorting, liquid penetrants, magnetic particle, microwave, thermal, and spark throwing. It can be seen that optical holography is one of many techniques which could be considered when a requirement arises in NDT.

Harwood[12] compares techniques which provide a picture of strain across the whole field of view, including photoelasticity, moire interferometry, laser holography, brittle lacquer, and SPATE (stress pattern analysis by thermal emission). Concerning holography, he concludes that "The technique requires complex and expensive equipment which must be set up exactly and completely isolated from extraneous inputs in order to give accurate data. Under ideal conditions the theoretical accuracy will be better than 1 μm... However, practical constraints mean that this high accuracy is unlikely to be achieved."

Kessler et al[13] compare the novel technique of scanning laser acoustic microscopy with ultrasonic testing, X-ray, fluorescent dye penetrant, destructive physical analysis, eddy current, and optical inspection (visual or microscopic). They give for each technique a brief description, its detection capability, and its advantages and disadvantages, as seen in Table II at the end of this paper.

Experimental comparison of holography, ultrasonics, and X-rays

Several pipe samples which had been examined holographically at Ontario Hydro were subsequently studied with ultrasonics and X-rays.

Eroded boiler tube

The furnace in a coal-fired generating station is lined with several banks of water filled boiler tubes which are exposed to the flame and fly ash. The tubes closest to the flame are subject to erosion and consequent wall thinning. Replacement programs for the tubes rely on a method of calculating residual life using spot checks, taken during routine shutdowns, on the remaining wall thickness of the tubes. The wall thickness is measured with an ultrasonic probe at normal incidence. In the past, it was necessary to grind off the scale and deposits which had built up on the surface before taking the measurements. However, a new instrument, the EMATS (ElectroMagnetic Acoustic Transducer) device, may obviate the need to remove the scale.

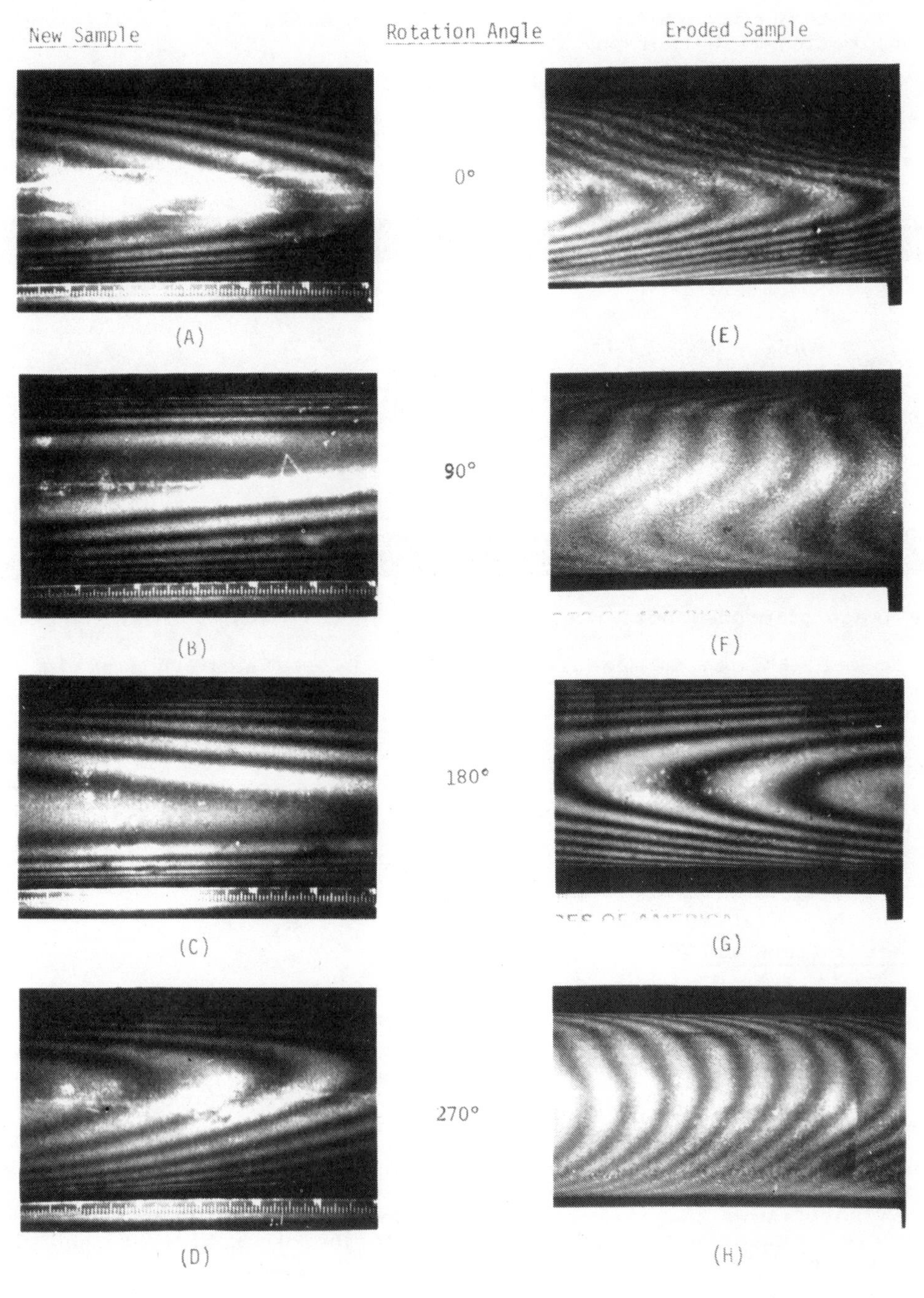

Fig. 11. Tubes exposed to flame in coal-fired boiler.

The rationale for a holographic approach was that a large area of tubing could be observed with one hologram, taken in a non-contact fashion so that a greater proportion of the tubes could be checked, perhaps even 100%. To implement this method in the field would require a means to accommodate vibration, to apply a suitable load, to compensate for rigid body motion, to eliminate the effects of air currents and heat waves, and to analyze and interpret a large number of interferograms.

Double exposure holographic interferograms were taken on both new and used boiler tube samples subjected to pressure. Rust and scale on the eroded tube were of no hindrance in taking the holograms; in fact the diffuse surface avoided glint and highlights. Fringes approximating the elliptical shape expected theoretically for an ideal tube were obtained on a sample of new tubing shown in the left column of Fig. 11. By contrast, an eroded sample cut from a section of tubing that had failed in service gave the pattern seen on the right in Fig. 11 where the fringes depart considerably from elliptical. In this sample, taken some distance from the failure site, the wall was thinned from 10 mm to 9 mm over 30% of the circumference, approximately.

It can be seen that holography easily detects 10% erosion over a wide area, making this a potential application of holography for NDT.

Figure 12 shows an X-ray image of the sample of used boiler tubing taken by a commercial inspection services company found in the Yellow Pages . This image did not readily show the wall thinning, an outcome expected by the X-ray technician. To use X-ray images for wall thickness measurement one can make quantitative measurements of the intensity.

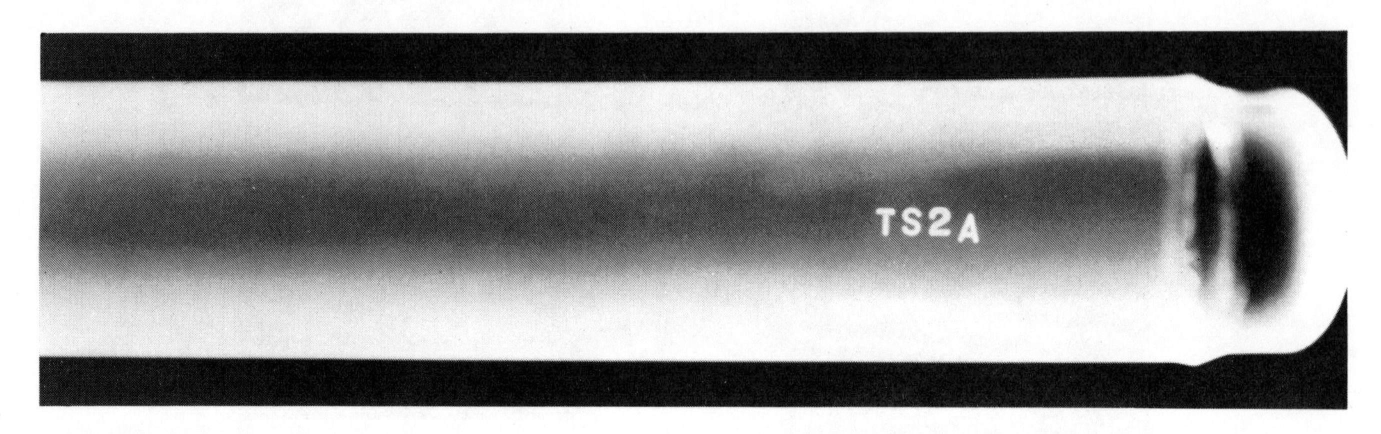

Fig. 12. X-ray image of eroded boiler tube does not show 10% wall thinning readily.

Ultrasonic wall thickness measurements were also taken with a small portable wall thickness meter with reliable results. There was a need to apply a liquid couplant and hold the probe in place by hand for each location probed.

Comparing holography, X-rays, and ultrasonics for evaluation of thermal plant boiler tubes, it could be inferred from the above that X-rays are not suitable for the detection of wall thinning unless quantitative image intensity measurements are taken. Ultrasonics are obviously suitable since this is the conventional method. Holography would appear to be an additional technique that could be used since it showed clear differences between new tubing and a tube that had failed in service.

Artificial defect in tube wall

Artificial defects in the form of slots 12 mm long and 0.4 mm wide were machined in the inside wall of a sample of 57 mm diameter steel tubing with a 3.9 mm thick wall. An axially oriented slot of depth 65% of wall thickness was formed in one side and a circumferential slot 23% deep was located on the other side, displaced somewhat axially. Figure 13 shows the results from three NDT techniques. A holographic interferogram obtained with a pressure change is shown in (a) for the side containing the axial slot. Approximately two fringes can be attributed to the slot, while the large scale fringe pattern represents the normal expansion. The tube sample was a low grade pipe apparently made by welding a spiral coil wound from flat stock. The overall fringe pattern is distorted from the expected pattern of ellipses and thereby shows the effects of wall nonuniformities. The more shallow circumferential slot was detectable in an interferogram of the other side of the tube as a slight distortion of the normal background fringe pattern.

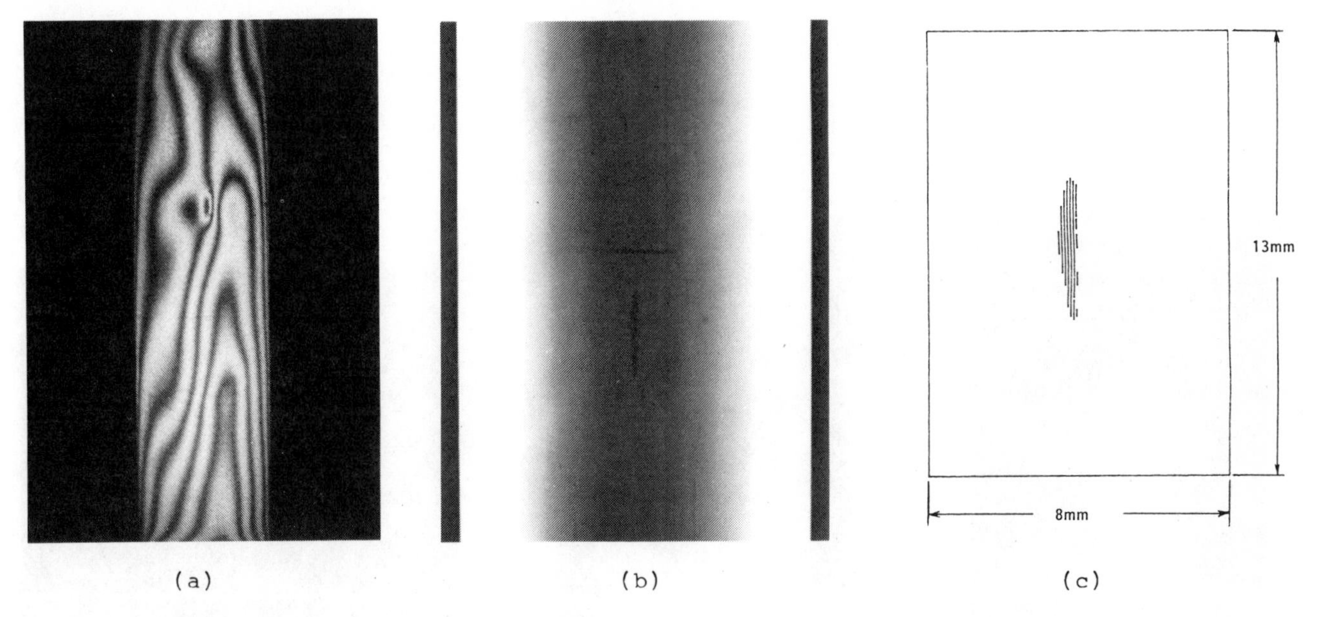

Fig. 13. Defect on inside wall of tube: (a) holographic interferogram with pressure change, (b) X-ray image clearly showed slots on both sides, on original film, (c) thresholded ultrasonic C-scan. Note that the three figures have different scale sizes.

An X-ray image is shown in Fig. 13 (b), taken straight through the pipe and revealing both slots. The slots were easily detected with just one exposure being taken by a skilled operator. The X-ray image accurately shows the location and length of the slots. The image is slightly blurred, yielding an overestimate of slot width. The depth of the slot can be inferred from the darkening of the film at the slot relative to that of the surrounding wall. This slot orientation, namely in a plane parallel to the direction of travel of the X-rays, is ideal for detection by X-rays.

An ultrasonic image of the axial slot is shown in Fig. 13(c), obtained by finding a suitable displaying threshold for a "C-scan" in which the amplitude of the reflected ultrasonic energy is observed. The image of the slot is shorter than the slot because the slot profile is elliptical leading to less reflected energy, below the threshold, toward the ends. The broadening of the image is due to the limitation on resolving power set by the wavelength of the ultrasonic waves being used.

All three methods were able to clearly show the 65% deep axial slot.

The ability of ultrasonics to obtain a quantitative measurement of slot depth is demonstrated in Fig. 14 which shows a "B-scan" across the slot. Here, the arrival time of the reflected wave is displayed and can be converted to distance travelled through the material, since the speed of the waves is known.

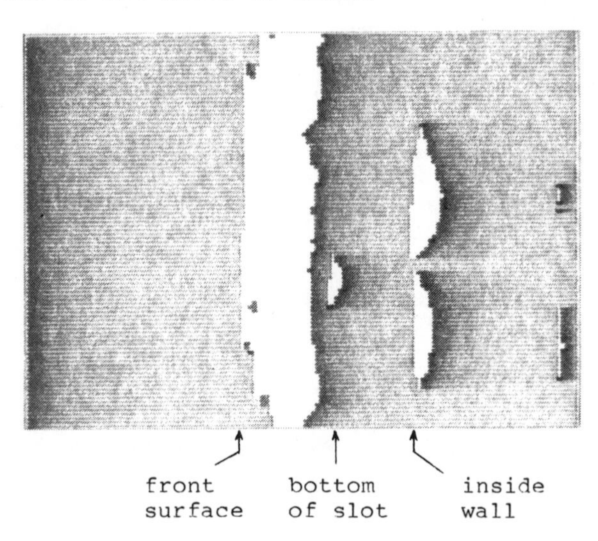

Fig. 14. Ultrasonic B-scan showing slot depth.

Steam reheater pipe with crack near end

A cracked tube removed from a boiler in a coal-fired power plant was examined holographically. The tube had been removed from service prior to failure thanks to an ultrasonic inservice inspection program. On the cut and polished end of the tube sample several hairline cracks with depths over half of the tube wall thickness were visible before a fixture was welded into the end to allow pressurization for holographic interferometry.

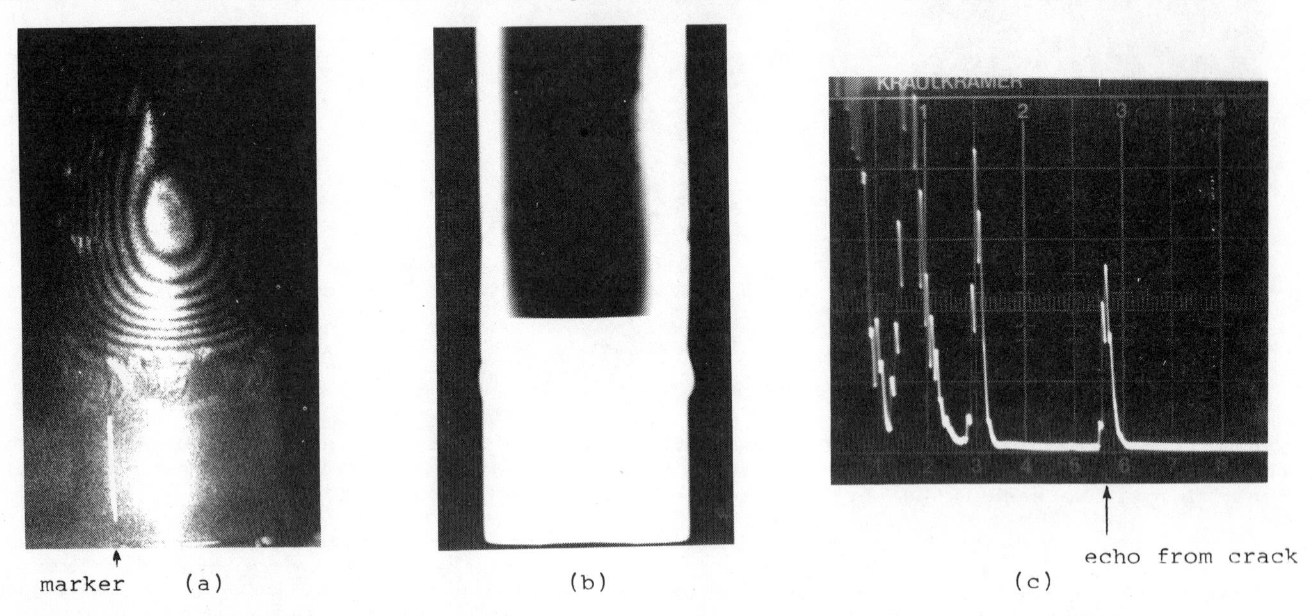

Fig. 15. Cracked reheater tube: (a) holography, (b) X-ray, (c) ultrasonic search.

Figure 15 shows the results of three techniques. A hairline crack about 80% of the way through the wall from the inside, whose location was marked on the outside as indicated in the figure, was not detected in either the holographic interferogram or in the X-ray image shown here, whereas the ultrasonic search seen in Fig. 15(c) clearly shows the presence of a crack. In defense of holography it should be noted that the plug welded into the end of the pipe for pressurization would reinforce the end where the cracks were and thereby reduce the effect of the cracks on pipe deformation. That is, crack detection would have been more probable had the cracks been located some distance from the end piece. In defense of the X-ray technique it will be admitted that only one X-ray was taken and that it was somewhat overexposed. Alternatively, the pressurization end piece which projected into the tube may have been too absorbing for the exposure used. It should be noted that both the X-ray and ultrasonic data shown above were taken after the sample had been fitted with the pressurization end pieces. Thus the ultrasonic result confirmed that welding in the end piece had not sealed up the cracks.

The above experience seems to cast doubt on the ability of holography (and X-rays) to detect hairline cracks, whereas the ultrasonic method gave a clear indication.

Acoustic holography

Acoustic holography grew out of the application of holographic imaging to ultrasonics. With the advent of high speed microcomputers, the computational method of data reduction and image creation has become practical. Hildebrand,[14] states "As with optical holography, selected applications (of acoustic holography) are beginning to find favor. A specific example is the use of ultrasonic holography for inspection of nuclear reactor pressure vessels." Further, he describes a commercial system which "...has been evaluated in the laboratory on flat and curved blocks, and on pipe samples with excellent results. One field trip to a nuclear power plant was also successful; in this case, indications in a girth weld of a steam generator shell were evaluated."

Vibration visualization and hologrammetry in nuclear plants

Tozer et al[15] have reported on a major effort to develop transportable equipment for field holography. With double pulse exposures, an in-service observation was made on a resonant vibration mode of a large bellows in the gas cooling duct of a Magnox nuclear power station. In hologrammetry, high resolution holograms are to be obtained on components inside reactors. Dimensional measurements may then be made on the real image at leisure in a non-radioactive environment.

New developments in holography

Compensation for rigid body motion in field holography. A recently published solution to the rigid body motion problem encountered when holographic interferograms are taken under field conditions is to mount the holographic plate on the object and make a Denisyuk hologram with a pulsed laser. A method for developing such holograms, and practical examples of NDT tests, are given by Van Renesse et al.[16]

Assessment of flaw severity. The conventional approach to estimation of flaw severity is first to measure the flaw size and then calculate the expected flaw growth rate using the methods of fracture mechanics. An alternative approach which is inherently better suited to inteferometry is described by Juptner et al,[17] for example, in which they obtain the stress intensity factor from holographic fringes emanating from the crack tip. Translations of the surface are measured along a line perpendicular to the crack.

Easier interpretation of fringe patterns. Higher detection sensitivity. Neumann[18] has demonstrated a method to subtract the phase terms between a master object and an object under test to show the difference. He claims that in holographic NDT this will highlight anomalies in the object under test. Since the spatial frequency is reduced, he states that the test stress may then be greatly increased to yield increased detection sensitivity.

Difficult Access. Gilbert et al[19] delivered illumination to the sample by means of an individual optical fiber and an image was brought out on a flexible imaging bundle of the sort used in borescopes and endoscopes. A good fringe pattern was obtained when the sample was mounted on the optical table with vibration isolation and was observed in air. With the sample immersed in water and/or not vibration isolated, the fringe quality was degraded, but was still usable. A need was seen for imaging fiber bundles to be less sensitive to bending and vibration than those presently made from multimode fibers. Bjelkhagen[20] gives a review of the use of optical fibers in holographic interferometry, with emphasis on pulsed laser techniques.

Ceramic Materials. Sciammarella[21] has used holographic interferometry to detect cracks as small as 50 μm in depth in ceramic materials.

New developments in nonholographic techniques

Improvemements are continually being made in a large number of NDT techniques including conventional and novel techniques such as holography. Illustrative examples are given in this section of advances in nonholographic techniques.

An important aspect of NDT is measuring the size of defects so that their severity can be assessed either through use of inspection codes or the theory of fracture mechanics. Clearly techniques which provide a true three-dimensional image of a flaw would require less interpretation than other techniques. Acoustic holography is one of several techniques to present ultrasonic data in image form. A synthetic aperture can be provided by a one-dimensional array and use of several frequencies. Hildebrand[14] claims that this technique, which responds to sharp variations, is the best ultrasonic method for imaging cracks.

Tomography provides radiography with a three-dimensional imaging capability. The radiation could be X-rays, or gamma rays from a radioactive source. Tonner and Tosello[22] have reported on the use of computer assisted tomography for sizing of shrink cavities in valve castings.

Detection reliability has been of concern in the past, even for ultrasonic NDT. Aaltio and Kauppinen,[23] for example, reported that detection probability rarely exceeded 60% for significant flaws in ultrasonic inspections. However, improvements in probes and in procedures have ensued from a large international program known as PISC[24] (Programme for the Inspection of Steel Components) in which detection probabilities of 90% have been achieved.

Lasers may be used to generate ultrasonic waves. They can generate surface acoustic waves to detect small surface or near-surface defects, according to Maldague et al.[25] In addition, Monchalin[26] has described laser systems for exciting and probing ultrasonic waves in test pieces at high temperature. The fine focusing ability of lasers leads to microscopy which may have applications in NDT discussed by Kessler et al.[13] A short duration laser pulse striking the surface of an object can produce an ultrasonic wave of higher frequency and shorter wavelength than the more conventional piezoelectric transducers. Hence, smaller defects can be detected and imaged. Since higher frequency waves are attenuated more, the technique is more suited to detection of defects close to the surface.

A miniature linear accelerator (MINAC) has been developed by Jones[27] to provide high energy X-rays in order to achieve greater penetration and shorter exposure times. These features improve the performance of the radiographic technique in the detection of intergranular stress corrosion cracking (IGSCC), a potential failure mechanism in boiling water reactors (BWRs). An experimental unit has been successfully used to evaluate components in a nuclear power plant. Such "high quality" radiography, while not as sensitive as ultrasonics, is considered to be a complementary technique which can provide confirmation of ultrasonic indications.

A problem with conventional ultrasonic testing is the need to provide a couplant between the transducer and the workpiece. EMAT testers, which need no couplant, have been used to inspect cladding tubes for nuclear fuel rods in the Federal Republic of Germany, as described by Gerhardt and Kayser.[28]

For inspection of tubes inside heat exchangers used in power generation facilities, Carodiskey and Meyer[29] have described an array of ultrasonic transducers for use instead of a spinning head.

Discussion and critical review - new directions for holographic NDT

The author is pleased to acknowledge discussions with several Ontario Hydro experts who are involved in NDT for power plants: J. Graham, K.S. Mahil, S. Buhay, J.A. Baron, M.P. Dolbey, J.D. Tulk, M.T. Flaman, N. Anyas-Weiss, S.M. Harvey and K.B. Woodall. The discussions are summarized in part below, with some of the conversational flavor left intact.

Screening test for conventional NDT

"It's not an either/or situation. You may find that you may want to do some preliminary wide-scale screening with holography and then go in with ultrasonics for precision measurements at certain locations."

Boiler tubes in coal-fired boilers. Although utilities can tolerate some failures of boiler tubes in coal plants, they want to guard against a rash of failures, especially in their peak season. Now, with spot checks they are liable to miss bad areas of tubing. What they need is a method to say, "That bank up there needs to be looked at now." This would be very valuable to them. "While the present method of measuring boiler tube wall thickness is ultrasonics, it is expensive because the scale has to be ground off, at least at the present time. Holography would be useful if it could look at large banks of water-wall tubes and at least pick out the thin ones from the thick ones in areas of erosion and corrosion. That would be a lot more efficient than doing spot checks with an ultrasonic probe. Certainly the potential is there for some real benefits if holography could be made to work."

Identification of high stress areas. A large flaw in a low stress area would not be as severe as a small flaw in a high stress area. Either one assumes the strain distribution in the components or one measures it with strain gages. "We spent $1 M at one nuclear power plant on strain gage measurements of stresses in pipe elbows, joins between pipes, and joins between pipes and large vessels." When the high stress areas have been identified, ultrasonic investigation, which is very time consuming, can be carried out in the areas most prone to failure.

Historical tracking. "I was reminded of vibration signature analysis when you were talking. In this technique you may get quite different signatures from components which are nominally the same. However the technique becomes useful when you take initial baseline signatures and then compare them with later results. This is valuable if you are able to interpret the changes in the signatures in terms of changes, either bad or benign, in the component. So with holography, you could also keep track of the fringe pattern of a given tube to see how it is changing with time. Ones that are changing rapidly would be cause for alarm."

"One use of holography that I can think of would be in checking systems that have to remain in alignment over a period of time."

Reformulation of design/build/certify philosophy

The present method of designing, building, and certifying pressure vessels is based in part on the presently accepted NDT techniques and their limitations. Since X-rays or ultrasonics can detect cracks, the design/build/certify philosophy is based on flaw detection rather than, say, response to pressure. Since X-rays and ultrasonics may not always be able to discriminate between flaws and the benign background clutter, a factor of safety is included in ASME[4] and other NDT code requirements. This means that the codes specify more stringent acceptance criteria than would be required if better NDT techniques were available. There are also safety factors included in the design phase, so that wall thicknesses may be specified to be greater than those that would be needed in a design/build/certify philosophy based on a fitness-for-service NDT method.

Concerning the pitting in the valve body studied by Doty and Hildebrand,[9] "you would probably find that it wasn't an especially damaging flaw. You would find you could drill a hole right through, tap it, put in a threaded plug, and find you still had a perfectly acceptable valve. From my understanding of fracture mechanics there may be some flaws like slag inclusions in welds which are not particularly damaging even though they are over 10%, whereas other sharp flaws like cracks can be relatively severe. One shouldn't base an evaluation scheme entirely on whether or not certain sized flaws or voids can be detected."

"The problem we have is that we build things conservatively. That valve could probably have been reduced 80% in wall thickness and still survived."

Again, "we build components to certain criteria which depend on our ability to test them in service and ensure that they are fit for service. Since flaw detection with conventional techniques is prone to error and uncertainty, we build conservatively. This means that when holography comes along, it is trying to find small flaws in rather rigid vessels with thick walls. It has a tough job, then, because surface deformations will be small."

"A point to remember is that conventional NDT techniques are time consuming to apply so it is not economical to apply them very often. Therefore we need plenty of advance warning when we rely on the conventional techniques. On the other hand, if we had a rapid technique which could be applied more often, we could tolerate later detection of deterioration, so that the flaw detection capability could be coarser."

Alternatively, components could be designed less conservatively if we were closer to a direct fitness-for-service testing technique. "Even for conventional NDT methods, overdesigning the components causes difficulty. Their performance on thick walled vessels (we have some up to 250 mm thick) is seriously in question."

Surface deformation as an NDT technique. A line of research would be to look at deformations in response to pressure in components with flaws and then test them to destruction to see if holography would have provided sufficient early warning on flaws which could in fact have caused the vessel to destroy itself. This sort of research could show whether the technique is capable of finding important flaws as opposed to merely finding a flaw of a specific size which may or may not present a danger to the vessel. Techniques which detect surface deformation in response to pressurization include non-contact methods such as holographic interferometry, moire, photoelasticity, and optical triangulation, as well as contact methods.

"An analogy would be the criterion for pulling over to the side of the road because your car engine is in trouble. Traditionally you drive it as long as the oil pressure is over some standard value, assuming that this ensures that your bearings won't overheat and seize up. But you could alternatively check bearing friction directly, and keep driving the car no matter what the oil pressure was, as long as the bearing friction was satisfactory."

This amounts to saying that flaw size is an indirect way of detecting whether or not a pressure vessel is in trouble. If you had a more direct way of checking what the vessel was doing, such as detecting deformation of the surface, you may have an NDT technique which directly gives a fitness-for-service indication. "I don't know if surface deformation would be a sufficient quantity to monitor, but it would be worth pursuing and doing some research on it."

It should be noted that one case where surface deformation did not appear to be sensitive enough was the cracked steam reheater pipe shown in Fig. 15 which was removed from service because ultrasonics had found cracks 80% of the way through the wall right at the end where the pipe was welded to a header. These probably were dangerous cracks, and holography did not detect them.

Complementary technique. "Holography and ultrasonics seem to be two complementary techniques. Ultrasonics responds to sharp discontinuities, while holography is better at soft discontinuities over a broad area, such as corrosion and erosion."

Improvement of signal-to-noise ratio

It would appear from the work of Martin,[7] for example, that holography is not sensitive enough to detect flaws of small enough size to serve the ASME scheme of vessel evaluation. However, several methods are available to increase the sensitivity of holography: heterodyning, shorter wavelengths, computers, etc. "So a one-fringe detection criterion is conservative and in fact you could actually detect much smaller flaws. Why do you limit yourself to the one-fringe criterion?"

"This is a question of signal-to-noise ratio. Any detection scheme must have a signal-to-noise ratio over 1 in order to make a detection. Often people discuss mainly the signal end of things, because it's difficult to assess the noise since it depends on the environment. Martin, for one, set his detection limit at one fringe, which means his resolving power was one fringe in his opinion."

"Another way to increase your signal would be to increase the pressure, because you were using pressures well under the maximum pressure you could have used. Why don't you increase the sensitivity by working at higher pressures?"

"Mainly because you get too many background fringes. The normal fringe pattern becomes so dense that the fringes become lost in the speckle. Part of your noise is speckle noise. Looking at Martin's photo in Fig. 6 you can see that the fringes at the edge of the pipe are already starting to blur together, though in the center you could indeed still see them at higher pressure."

"So you could rotate the pipe and look at the center region of it, strip by strip, with higher pressure and therefore higher signal-to-noise ratio."

"Yes, this would help to discriminate against environmental effects such as vibration and heat waves. Also, you could turn to the comparative technique of Neumann.[18]"

For any NDT technique, a flaw can be detected only if the signal to noise ratio, after all processing has been done, is greater than one. Noise consists of random fluctuations and systematic errors. In ultrasonics, for example, the small amount of random noise present in the signal amplifiers is generally insignificant in comparison to systematic errors in the form of extraneous reflections from benign interfaces such as that between the base metal and the cladding on the inside of pressure vessels.

Similarly in holography it is important to recognize that there may be significant sources of noise in addition to quantum shot noise. Wagner,[30] for instance, found his noise was an order of magnitude greater than expected on the basis of shot noise. He speculated that the additional noise was due to his detectors and amplifiers, and due to variation in pathlength owing to environmental effects. He also calculated that speckle would introduce five times more uncertainty into his measurements than shot noise. Since his experiment was on a flat two-dimensional plate where there was no need to trade off small speckle size to achieve sufficient depth of field, greater speckle noise would be expected in observations on three-dimensional objects.

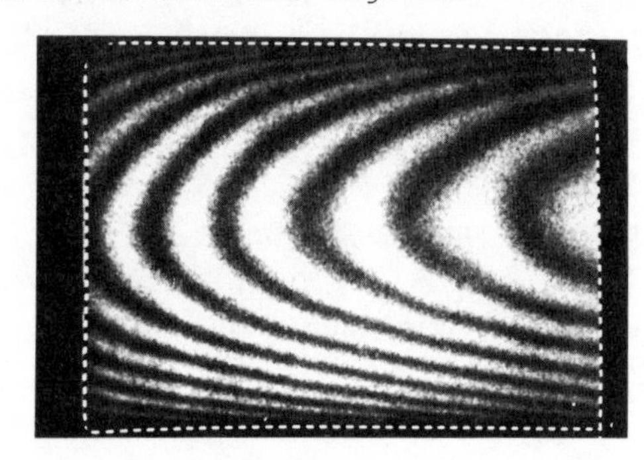

(a) Raw data

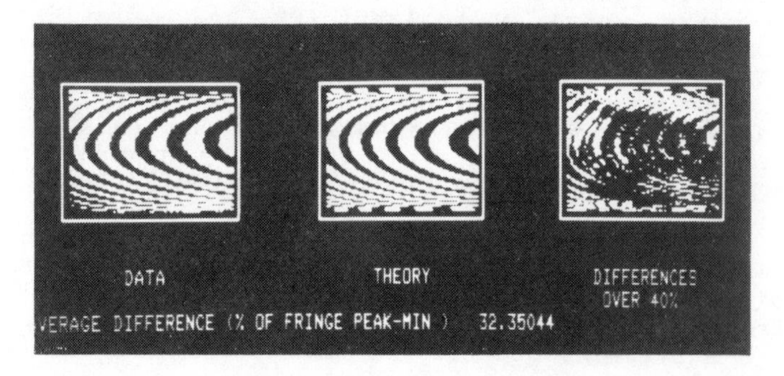

(b) Quantitative analysis

Fig. 16. Heat waves can distort fringes and lead to false alarms on the presence of flaws. Areas of misfit between the processed data and theory for an ideal tube show up on the difference plot in (b). Here the misfit is due to heat waves, not flaws. Source: Mader.

Mader[1] found disturbances of about half a fringe over a broad region due to heat waves (index of refraction variations) in the interferogram seen in Fig. 16 of a tube heated 5.4°C. The integration time was that of a video frame grabber, 1/30 s, from which the severity of the disturbance could be estimated for different exposure times. Assuming a square root dependence in the statistics, then averaging over 256 frames, for example, would reduce the effect from half of a fringe to 1/32 of a fringe. The disturbance was known to be due to heat waves and not a flaw because the interferogram had been viewed in real-time. Had this been a double exposure hologram, no such knowledge would have been available. A comparison of the bends in the fringes in Fig. 16 with those seen in Fig. 11 (H) for an eroded tube shows that heat waves could produce distortions similar to pipe defects so that the heat waves cannot be filtered out without losing some information about flaws. To reduce the effect of heat waves, then, the object should be at room temperature or should be in a vacuum chamber. The exposure time should be long to average over the fluctuations in the convection currents, and of course the apparatus should be enclosed to avoid room air currents due to air conditioners or the movement of people. These considerations become a challenge to implement in the field.

Turning to systematic errors, the complexity of the normal fringe pattern for an unflawed component can cause confusion in fringe pattern interpretation, as seen by Doty and Hildebrand,[9] for example, in their experiment on a valve. The distortion of fringes due to heat waves could also be classified as a systematic error since such distortion can easily mimic the effect of small or deeply buried flaws that introduce less than one extra fringe.

Information available on flaw size in interferograms

Optical holography provides a means to observe and measure, for points on the surface of solid objects, the displacement caused by application of a test load. For the detection of flaws it is necessary to detect the difference in surface displacement between a normal sample and a flawed sample. In principle, even deeply buried flaws can produce measurable effects at the surface, though their effect at the surface diminishes rapidly with their depth. (X-rays penetrate the object and so are equally sensitive to voids wherever they occur within the body of the object.) When several flaws are present, their surface effects are likely to blend together and make interpretation difficult. The fundamental consideration from an information theory point of view is the dimensionality. First, the information we are attempting to obtain is three-dimensional, namely, the location and size of three-dimensional flaws scattered throughout a three-dimensional solid. Second, optical holography gives us access only to a surface, which is inherently two-dimensional. Thus, fundamental progress in holographic NDT can occur only if the NDT problem can be reformulated such that sufficient information to ensure that an object is fit for service can be obtained from observations of a two-dimensional nature. The work of Juptner et al, for example, to obtain the stress intensity factor and to relate this to strength is part of such a reformulation.

Comments on a niche for holographic NDT for defect detection

Why is holography one of the preferred methods for detection of defects in aircraft tires and honeycomb panels? Among the several reasons, one could cite material properties, test requirements, and dimensionality of the problem. On material properties, tire testing presents a number of obstacles to conventional NDT. Ultrasonic waves would suffer severe attenuation in rubber and would also be scattered and reflected by the normal reinforcing belts. Considering the test requirements, the flaws to be detected are generally delaminations between the tire carcass and the tread. X-rays would be inherently unsuited to detect such flaws since the flaws are broadside to the direction of X-ray propagation. Such flaws, being buried flaws, are of course inaccessible to surface flaw detection techniques. Similar considerations would eliminate essentially all nonholographic NDT techniques. Holography, however, is suited to tire testing. The material has a low value of Young's modulus, so that a pressure load of only one atmosphere (applied negatively as a vacuum) is sufficient. Since the flaws are internal and are sealed (no surface breaking cracks are involved), and since the vacuum is applied to both inside and outside of the tire, the background fringe pattern is minimal. This reduces the clutter of normal fringes, thus improving the signal (fringes due to flaws) to background ratio. Since the test environment is a vacuum chamber, interference from air currents is eliminated. Since the tires are easily removed from the vehicle or aircraft for inspection and are of a relatively small size, they can be tested under laboratory conditions conducive to successful application of interferometry.

Aluminium honeycomb panels for aircraft are also routinely tested with holography for debonds between the skin and the honeycomb structure. Although Young's modulus is much higher than for rubber, the loads needed to produce sufficient surface deflection are small because the skin is thin for light weight. Since debonds are obviously close to the surface they have a relatively large effect on surface displacement. This, coupled with the inherently rigid nature of the panels, leads to a large number of fringes due to the flaws, seen against a background of relatively few fringes. Thus holography provides a high signal to noise ratio. Nonholographic techniques, on the other hand, are plagued with small signals in the case of X-rays, or a confusing background in the case of ultrasonics.

The dimensionality of the problem in both tire testing and honeycomb panels is suited to holography. The delaminations in one case and the debonds in the other case occur essentially in a known plane parallel to the surface within the body of the object . That is, the flaws are not three-dimensional defects scattered throughout the volume of the component. Rather, in these two successful applications of holography, the flaws are two-dimensional as befits an NDT technique that examines the two-dimensional surface of the component.

The above discussion leads to the following guidelines for a search for further applications for holographic NDT as applied to defect detection:

1. Holographic NDT should have advantages over nonholographic NDT techniques.
2. Materials or components should be sought where nonholographic techniques suffer from low signal or high noise and background clutter.

3. Components which can be tested in a laboratory-type environment should be sought.

4. A differential technique for holography should be sought where fringes are produced only by the presence of flaws, such as evacuation of both the inside and outside of tires or comparative holography.

5. Flat two-dimensional flaws lying in a plane parallel to the surface are of the correct dimensionality for optical holography. Broad areas of wall thinning would also have the correct dimensionality.

One example which fulfills some of the above points is detection of broad areas of corrosion or erosion in the wall of pressure vessels or pipes.

Conclusions

Holography is being used on a trial basis in support of power plants. Laboratory observations have been made to validate repair procedures by showing that they did not deform the part under repair.

In field work in nuclear power plants, acoustic holography has been used successfully to evaluate indications in a girth weld. Optical holography has been used in Magnox reactors for hologrammetry to take dimensional measurements to monitor deterioration of fuel bundles. Vibration fields have been observed for resonant vibration modes on a large bellows.

Detection of defects in the field using holographic interferometry is at the study stage. Studies have been done at several laboratories on the ability of holography to detect defects of various types including voids and cracks. Methods for transferring holography to the field have been proposed including techniques to overcome rigid body motion and vibration.

In quantitative studies of sensitivity, the expected surface deformation (and its effect on the fringe pattern) due to a defect has been obtained for a limited number of single defect cases. Cracks on the inside wall away from end effects, simulated by short slots, were easily detectable provided their depth was over half of the wall thickness. The limit of detectability appears to be about 12% using a detection criterion of one fringe which is perhaps as good as could be expected in the field environment. This does not compare favorably with ASME[4] requirements of 3 to 12%. Pitting, simulated by drilling a blind hole, was detectable only for relatively large, deep pits.

Multiple defects have not been analyzed for their combined effect on an interferogram, leaving questions of fringe pattern analysis in such cases unanswered. It could be speculated, however, that there could be cases where, for example, several small flaws would give essentially the same fringe pattern as one larger flaw. If this could in fact happen it would be clear that optical holography, or any other method based on surface displacement, would be incapable of measuring defect sizes. Then, when considering acceptance or rejection of a flawed component, it would be necessary to change the criterion from defect size to surface deformation due to pressurization.

It is suggested that a deformation based approach to pressure vessel and pipe integrity be considered along with the present flaw based approach. The theoretical and historical correlations between deformation and vessel failure should be investigated along with suitable methods for field measurement of deformation. Such methods may include optical holography or other techniques.

For field work with holography, compensation is needed for limitations due to its fundamental properties:

(a) It is interferometric and therefore is prone to disturbance by vibration.

(b) Since it is noncontacting and since the intervening air has optical properties it responds to heat waves and air currents.

While advances are being made in holographic NDT, advances are also being made in other techniques, so that holography is unlikely to supplant them in applications where they have specific strengths, especially in a flaw based method of vessel evaluation. Holography will find a role in areas where conventional techniques have limitations and where holography has advantages in cost or technical performance. It is speculated that screening tests for corrosion or erosion may be one such area. To extend the use of holography to evaluation of pressure vessel and pipe integrity would likely require a shift from the present flaw based approach to one based on surface deformation.

References

1. Mader, D.L., "Holographic interferometry on pipes - precision interpretation by least-squares fitting", Appl. Opt., 24(22), 3784 (1985).

2. Hsu,T.R., "Computational Efficiency of FAXMOD and Development of Holo-camera for Fast Sheath Deformation Measurement," Thermomechanics Lab. Rep. No. 80-1-69, Univ. of Manitoba (1980).

3. Vest, C.M., "Status and Future of Holographic Nondestructive Evaluation", Holographic Nondestructive Testing, J. Ebbeni, ed., Proc. SPIE 349, 186 (1982).

4. ASME Boiler and Pressure Vessel Committee, ASME Boiler and Pressure Vessel Code, An American National Standard, Section XI: Rules for Inservice Inspection of Nuclear Power Plant Components, 1983 Edition, The American Society of Mechanical Engineers, New York (1983).

5. Copeland,J.F. and P.C. Riccardella, "The application of fracture mechanics leak-before-break analyses for protection against pipe rupture in SEP plants," in Proc. CSNI Specialist Meeting on Leak-Before-Break in Nuclear Reactor Piping, 468, U.S. Nuclear Regulatory Commission report NUREG/CP-0051 (1984).

6. Katzir, Y., A.A. Friesem, I. Glaser, B. Sharon, "Holographic nondestructive evaluation with on-line acquisition and processing," in Industrial and Commercial Applications of Holography, M. Chang, ed., Proc. SPIE 353, 74 (1983).

7. Martin, D.J.V., "Laser holographic and speckle photography methods for defect detection and strain evaluation in pressure vessels", in Nuclear Engineering and Design, Vol. 43, C.F. Bonilla and T.A. Jaeger, eds., 227, North-Holland Publishing Company, Amsterdam (1977). Also: Journal of Strain Analysis, 10(3), 143 (1975). Also: in Structural Mechanics in Reactor Technology, Vol. 3, Part G-H, T.A. Jaeger, ed., Chap. G 3/10, North-Holland Publishing Co., Amsterdam (1975).

8. Wachutka, H., H. Kordisch and B. Fischer, "Holographisch-Interferometrische Verformungsmessungen zur Bewertung lokaler Inhomogenitaten im Inneren dickwandiger Bauteile," VDI-Berichte Nr. 366 (1980).

9. Doty, J.L. and B.P. Hildebrand, "The Use of Sandwich Hologram Interferometry for Nondestructive Testing of Nuclear Reactor Components," Opt. Eng., 21(3), 542 (1982).

10. Roark, R.J. and W.C. Young, Formulas for Stress and Strain, 5th Ed., McGraw-Hill Book Co., New York (1975).

11. Boyer, Howard E., ed., Metals Handbook, Vol. 11: Nondestructive Inspection and Quality Control, American Society for Metals, Metals Park, Ohio (1976).

12. Harwood, N., "Relative assessment of full field experimental stress analysis techniques", Strain (Journal of the British Society for Strain Measurement) 21(3), 119 (1985).

13. Kessler, L.W., J.E. Semmens, F. Agramonte, "Scanning Laser Microscopy (SLAM): A New Tool for NDT", WCNDT*, p.995. Also: L.W. Kessler, IEEE Trans. on Sonics and Ultrasonics SU-32(2), 136 (1985).

14. Hildebrand, B.P., "Stepped Frequency Ultrasonic Holography for Flaw Characterization", WCNDT*, p.971. Also: "Progress in Acoustic Holography," in Holography, Lloyd Huff, ed., Proc. SPIE 532, 63 (1985).

15. Tozer,B.A., R. Glannville, A.L. Gordon, M.J. Little, J.M. Webster and D.G. Wright, "Holography applied to inspection and mensuration in an industrial environment," Applications of Holography, Lloyd Huff, ed., Proc. SPIE 523, 119 (1985). Also: Opt. Eng., 24(5), 746 (1985).

16. Van Renesse, R.L., and J.W. Burgmeijer, "Application of pulsed reflection holography to material testing," Opt. Eng. 24(6), 1086 (1985).

17. Juptner,W., K. Grunewald, R. Zirn, H. Kreitlow, "Measurement of the stress intensity factor K_I in large specimens by means of holographic interferometry", in Holographic Data Nondestructive Testing, Dalibor Vukicevic, ed., Proc. SPIE 370, 62 (1982).

18. Neumann, D.B., "Comparative holography: a technique for eliminating background fringes in holographic interferometry," Opt. Eng., 24(4), 625 (1985).

19. Gilbert,J.A., T.D. Dudderar and A.Nose, "Remote deformation field measurement through different media using fiber optics," Opt. Eng., 24(4), 628 (1985).

20. Bjelkhagen, H.I., "Pulsed fiber holography: a new technique for hologram interferometry", Opt. Eng. 24(4), 645 (1985).

21. Sciammarella, C.A., "Advances in the application of holography for NDE," in Applications of Holography, Lloyd Huff, ed., Proc. SPIE 523, 137 (1985).

22. Tonner, P.D. and G. Tosello, "An industrial application of computer assisted tomography: detection, location and sizing of shrink cavities in valve castings," Chalk River Nuclear Laboratories report AECL-8626, presented at the 5th Canadian Conference on Nondestructive Testing, Toronto, Oct. 28-31, 1984.

23. Aaltio, M. and Kauppinen, K.P., "Reliability and Defect Sizing," in Periodic Inspection Of Pressurized Components,I Mech E Conference Publications 1982-9, 283, Mechanical Engineering Publications Limited, London (1982).

24. PISC, "Pisc II probes NDE capabilities," Nuclear Engineering International, 30(375), 13 (1985).

25. Maldague, X., P. Cielo and C.K. Jen, "NDT Applications of Laser-Generated Focused Acoustic Waves", WCNDT*, p.784.

26. Monchalin, J., "Optical Detection of Ultrasound at a Distance by Laser Interferometry", WCNDT*, p.1017.
27. Jones, J.A., Applied Research Company, "IGSCC Detection in BWR Piping using the Minac," Electric Power Research Institute report EPRI NP-3828 (1985).
28. Gerhardt,R. and W. Kayser in "Concepts of NDT System Families for Industrial Applications", WCNDT*, p.730.
29. Carodiskey, T.J. and P.A. Meyer, "A Boreside Array - Its Design and Application", WCNDT*, p.760.
30. Wagner, J.W., "Heterodyne Holography for Visualization of Surface Acoustic Waves," in WCNDT*, p.1009.

* WCNDT = WCNDT, 11th World Conference on Nondestructive Testing 1985, Volume Two, by The World Conference on Nondestructive Testing, Taylor Publishing Co., Dallas (1985).

Table II. Comparison of nonholographic NDT techniques.
(This table adapted from Kessler et al)

Technique	Description	Detection	Advantages	Disadvantages
SLAM Scanning Laser Acoustic Micros-copy	High frequency (10-500 MHz) ultrasound images are produced in real-time using CW transducer and a scanning laser detector.	Image of internal volume is produced. Detects cracks, voids, porosity, and subsurface defects.	Rapid defect location and characterization. Accommodates complex shapes. Ideal for bond evaluation.	Sample must be immersed in fluid for ultrasonic coupling. Excessive porosity or struc-ture may mask flaws.
ULTRASONIC TESTING	Pulsed energy (1-25 MHz.) Focused transducer for transmitter and receiver.	Same as above.	Good penetration. Can select specific echoes for display.	Same as above, plus lower resolutuion, hard to scan complex geometries. Slow process.
X-RAY	X-rays are absorbed by material before exposing film.	Images show variations in in density due to wall thickness and defects.	Easy to use.	Long exposure time for thick specimens. Safety precautions needed. Must be adequate density difference to see defect.
FLOURES-CENT DYE PENETRANT	Sample is immer-sed in dye solution which seeps into fine cracks. Excess dye is removed.	Under UV light, fine cracks are visible, espe-cially with microscope.	Very sensitive for detecting defects which are difficult to observe.	Dye may leave contamination on surface. Can find only defects which are open to surface.
EDDY CURRENT	Measures impedance of probe coil,which depends on conduc-tivity of adjacent material.	Identifies foreign material, surface finish and surface discontinuity.	Easy to use on production line, and in the field.	Can only be used on metals. Quantitative measurement difficult.
VISUAL INSPECTION	Direct vision, or with magnifi-cation. Could use computer vision assistance.	Detects surface condition: burns, deposits, cracks, burrs, etc.	Universally applicable. Obtains precise location of defect.	Only surface defects detectable. Hard to computerize. Depends on operator judgement.

Holographic inspection of composites

John W. Newman

Laser Technology, Inc.
1055 W. Germantown Pike, Norristown, Pennsylvania 19403

Abstract

Holographic interferometry has developed into a powerful tool for the inspection of composite structures both at the manufacturing level in factory environments, as well as in damage assessment of aircraft in the field. Once performed only in the laboratory, holographic inspection is the preferred testing technology for certain bonded aircraft engine components. Holographic inspection applications of various composite structures are shown and test results presented.

Introduction

Until 1975 most holograms were produced on glass photographic plates using standard darkroom techniques for processing. Often, the processing of the hologram required 5 to 10 minutes at a cost per shot that was unacceptable for high production holographic inspection. The development of instant push-button hologram recording systems based on silver halide and thermoplastic film has lead to the implementation of production equipment which produce holograms in less than a minute for less than .25 cents each. In many cases, the hologram is presented to an inspector on a video monitor for evaluation seconds after the holographic exposure. Operator training of today's production holography equipment is limited to machine operation and evaluation of the video image. In certain applications in the aircraft engine industry, a production through-put of 200 parts on 1500 holograms per day has been achieved.

Every successful nondestructive testing system must achieve a defect sensitivity in test parts that is both repeatable and cost effective. In general, all NDT systems must meet the following criteria:

1. Ease of use with a minimum of operator/training.
2. Traceability of 100% between test result and part, both during evaluation of the test result and in the archival storage of the test result.
3. Repeatability of test result.
4. Ease of interpretation of test result.
5. Elimination of effect of environmental parameters on changes in test results.

The development of the automatic hologram recording system went a long way to improve the "ease of use", and the archival storage capability of the test result. The development of new techniques for stressing the test object during holographic inspection have improved test repeatability and eliminated the complexities involved in fringe line interpretation. In addition, new techniques for making holograms have greatly reduced the vibration isolation requirements.

Holographic recording systems

The elimination of glass photographic plate processing from the holographic inspection process has been instrumental in reducing both the material cost of holography as well as labor. Instant film processing uses a monobath solution in a microprocessor controlled camera using 35mm roll film. Not only are holograms produced in 10 seconds, but they may be reconstructed for real time viewing of test part deformation. At the press of a button, the film is advanced to a small exposure/processing chamber. The chamber is pressurized with water, wetting the emulsion and stabilizing the film during the exposure. After the holographic exposure, the monobath developer is pumped into the chamber, processing the film in-place. After the development process, water is pumped back into the chamber and the hologram is reconstructed with the reference beam. The image of the hologram is viewed by a video camera and presented to the operator some 10-15 seconds after the holographic exposure. Holograms made with this equipment are permanent and provide an archival record of the holographic inspection critical for NDE applications. The technique requires only 14 seconds for the entire film processing cycle. Refraction efficiencies of 7% are achieved with a reference to object beam intensity ratio of 4 to 1.

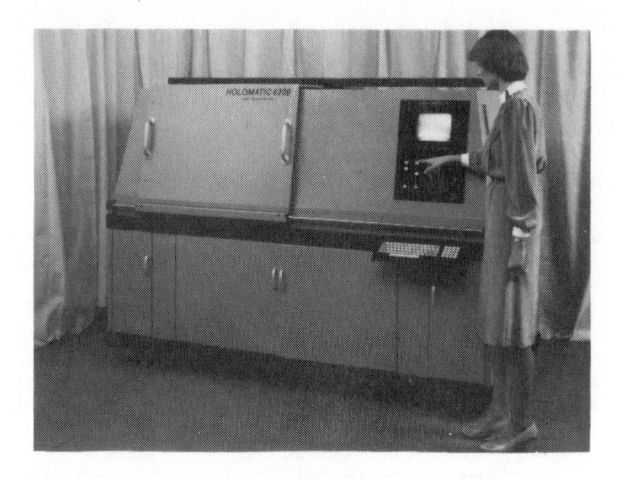

Figure 1. The HOLOMATIC 6200 Inspection System used to inspect bonded turbine engine components using holographic techniques. Up to 1500 holograms a day may be processed and evaluated.

Test part stressing techniques

The key to successful holographic inspection, after the holographic technique is automated and the cost reduced to an acceptable level, is the selection of the correct stressing technique to cause subsurface flaws to affect a localized surface deformation greater than one-half of the wavelength of the laser.

Single frequency versus white noise excitation

In the past, single exposure holograms were made while inducing a single frequency mechanical vibration into the test part.[1] Single frequency excitation of composite structures is seen in the time average hologram as an array of mode shapes and patterns reflecting those areas on the panel that are in vibration at that frequency. In general, unbonded areas in structures respond to a wider bandwidth of frequencies than does the structure itself. Fig. 2 shows an aluminum honeycomb panel containing unbonds, vibrating at 12,500 Hz. The unbonds are visible as small clusters of modal patterns and are not easily discerned. The development of coupled white noise vibration excitation by Claraday[2] has lead to a dramatic improvement in defect definition and sensitivity of holographic NDT. Fig. 3 shows the same honeycomb panel with the unbonds clearly defined as darkened areas on the face of the clearly seen panel. These dark areas are moving more than 1/2 the laser wavelength during the time average holographic exposure. The white noise vibration is exciting the part with frequencies between 15,000 and 25,000 Hz. simultaneously yielding an image identical to the result obtained using ultrasonic techniques. The test was performed in 15 seconds, however, instead of many minutes required by ultrasonics.

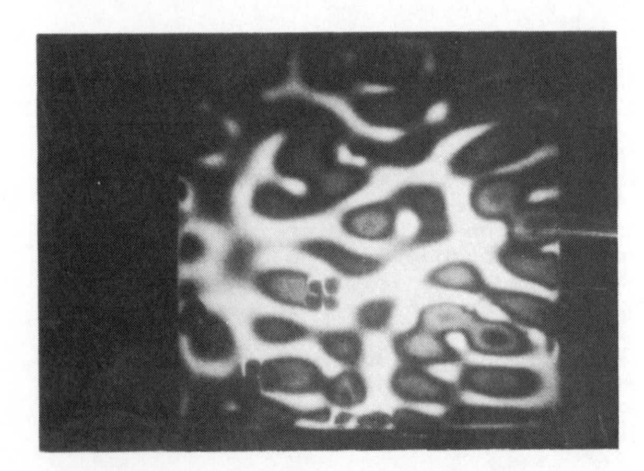

Figure 2. A 2 X 2 ft. Aluminum honeycomb panel vibrated at 12,250 Hz. During a time average hologram.

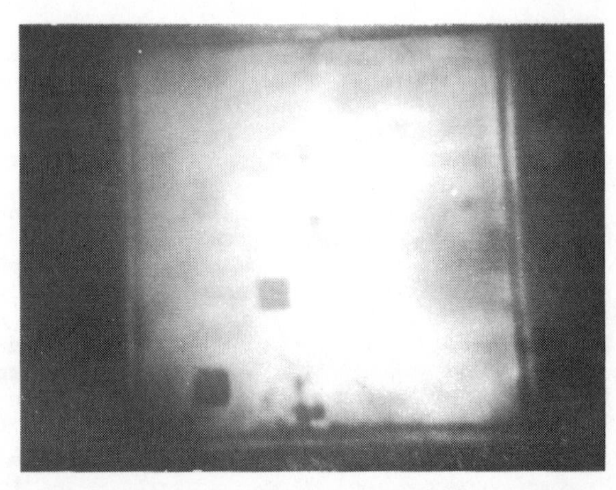

Figure 3. Same Aluminum panel tested with white noise excitation. Defects are clearly visible as dark areas.

Honeycomb panels with facesheet thickness less than 1/4 of the cell diameter may be easily excited with white noise to reveal not only unbonds but the distribution of bonding materials and single cell walls in the honeycomb as seen in the holographic test of the aluminum noise suppressor panel from a jet engine in Figures 4 and 5.

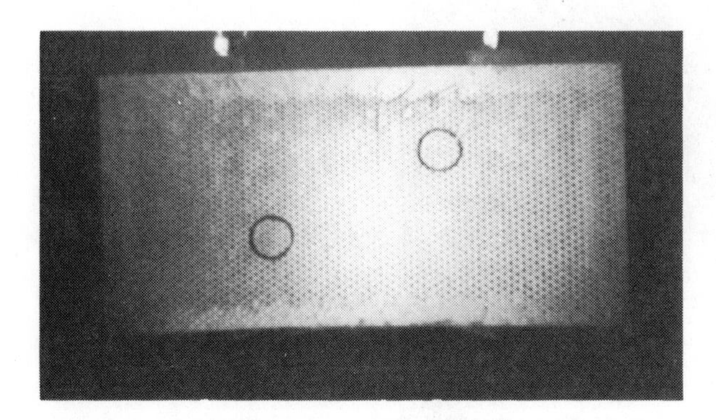

Figure 4. An aluminum honeycomb noise suppression panel from a jet engine. Note the perforated face sheet.

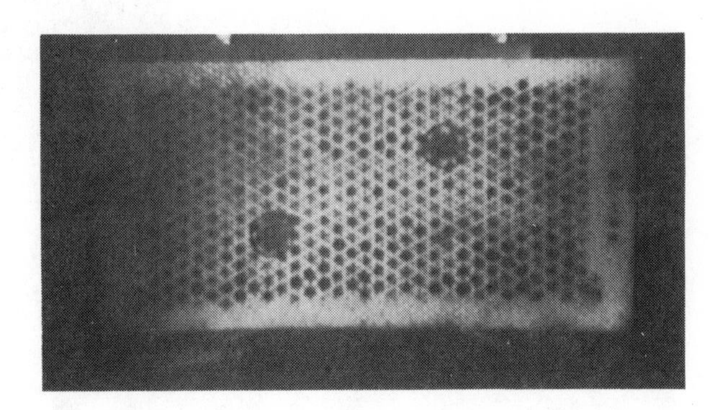

Figure 5. The holographic test of the panel shows individual honeycomb cells and and unbonds. Small facesheet perforations appear as small dots.

White noise excitation has proven to be invaluable to the application of holographic NDT to metallic bonded structures. The open cell steel honeycomb seal from an aircraft engine is easily inspected for honeycomb-to-backing ring unbonds as seen in Figures 6 and 7.

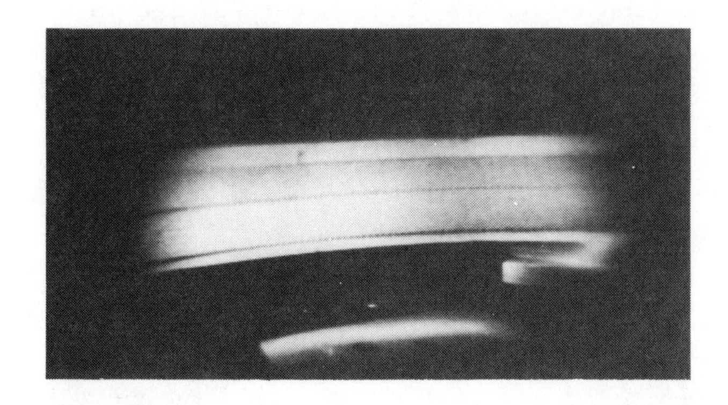

Figure 6. Open cell honeycomb seal from a PW JT-9D aircraft engine. Holographic inspection shows no unbonds.

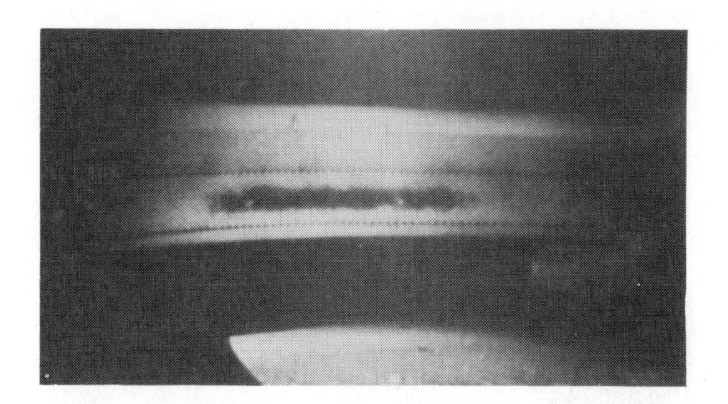

Figure 7. Another area on the same part showing an unbond measuring 7 inches in length.

Detecting moisture in composites with microwave excitation

In many airborne applications of honeycomb and composites structures, the detection of moisture is critical to the serviceability of the aircraft. Moisture is very difficult to detect with radiography, ultrasonics or eddy current inspection techniques presently used in aircraft maintenance.

Figure 8 shows the resulting time average hologram made of a graphite and Nomex core honeycomb panel containing several cells with water. During the holographic exposure, a microwave generator tuned to the excitation wavelength of the water was directed towards the panel heating the water. The slight temperature change caused a deformation of the surface in the facesheet immediately above the cells containing the water.

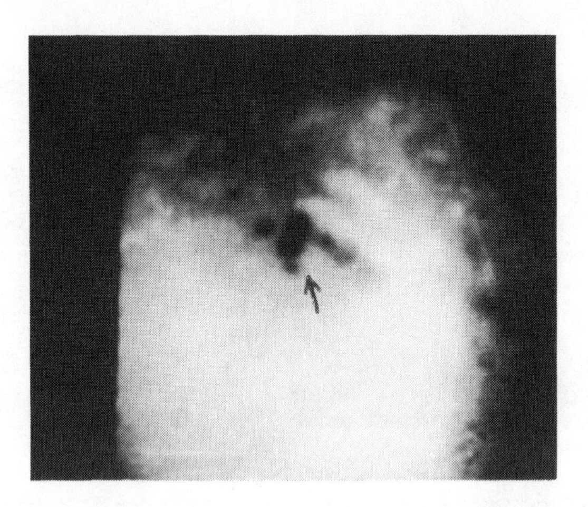

Figure 8. Time average hologram with microwave excitation reveals water filled cells in graphite/Nomex honeycomb panel.

Thermal testing of composites

Thermal stressing has been used in conjunction with double exposure holography for many years. The use of the automatic film processor has allowed the combination of thermal stressing with real-time holography, thermal stressing is applied between two holographic exposures. By trial and error, the correct heat load and times are developed for a given test part, a process requiring considerable time when using a glass photographic plates. With real-time holography, the hologram is made and processed. While the real-time image is being displayed, the heat may be judiciously applied to obtain the correct results in the first exposure.

Thermal loading is applicable to the detection of unbonds in honeycomb as well as to voids and delaminations in graphite structures and impact damage.

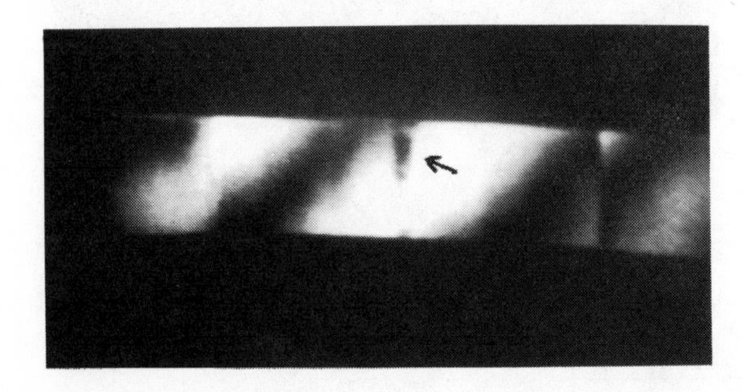

Figure 9. A Teflon strip embedded in a 1/2 inch graphite bar. Arrow points to the real-time image of the defect location.

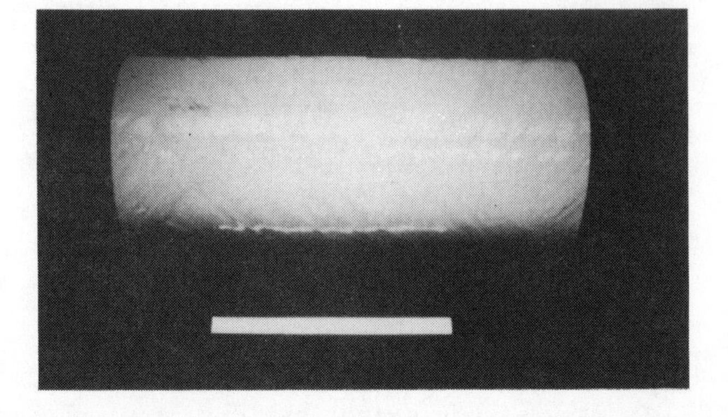

Figure 10. A filament wound tube with a 6 inch diameter and 3/8 inch wall thickness.

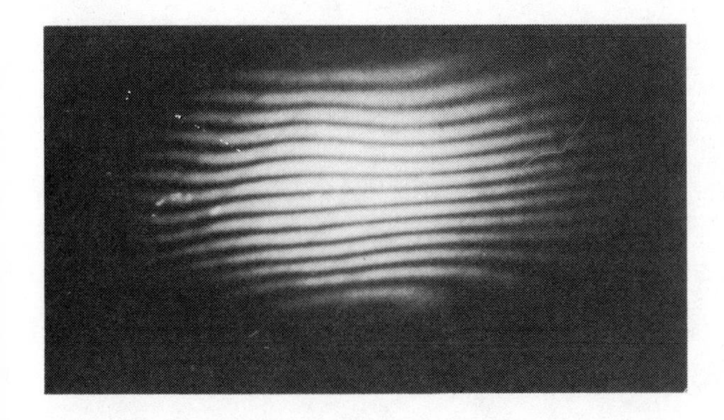

Figure 11. Defect free area on the tube as seen with real-time holographic inspection with thermal load.

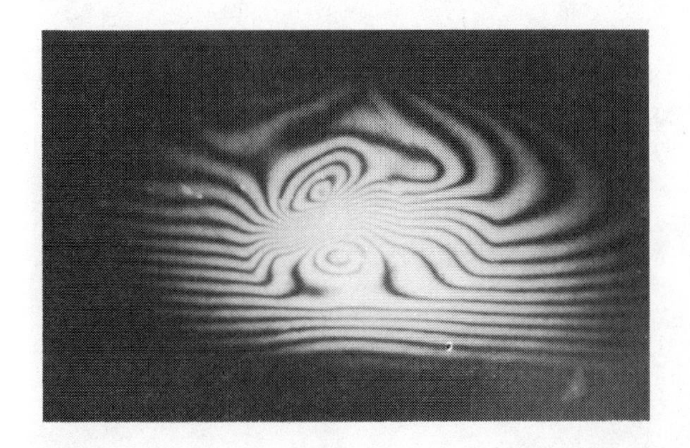

Figure 12. Same defect free area but tested after a small impact. Impact load was 1.2 ft. lbs. of force. Broken fibers are seen several inches away from the site of the impact.

Vacuum stressing of honeycomb panels

The technique of placing honeycomb panels in a reduced pressure atmosphere is well known in literature[3]. Double exposure and real-time holographic inspection with a vacuum pressure differential after the first exposure still leaves the defect in an array of displacement with fringe lines making interpretation and defect resolution difficult. A time average hologram with a small pulsing pressure change induces a motion in the facesheet above the unbond greater than 1/2 of the wavelength of the laser yielding test results similar to white noise vibration excitation.

Phase locked holography for holographic inspection in the field

Holography requires the stability of the interference pattern between the object and the reference beams to at least 1/4 of the wavelength of the laser during the exposure time. Usually, with CW lasers this requires a vibration isolation table for mounting the optical components, or the elimination of the beam splitter and most of the usual optical components in a basement laboratory using techniques developed by Abramson[4].

Over the last six months, the author's team has developed a phase locked holographic system. Using a 35mw HeNe laser, the path length difference between the object beam and the reference beam is measured and corrected for a near zero phase difference. This reduces the vibration requirements of the holographic system to the point where it may be tripod mounted and portable.

Using real time holography, two studies were made demonstrating the capabilities of the phase locked holography approach. A hologram was made of a cinderblock wall. An area of 5 sq. ft. was shot using a 20 second exposure. The hologram was processed in-place and reconstructed in real-time. It was discovered that the cinder blocks in the wall could be moved with the press of a finger and that they appear to move independently. Figure 13 shows the real time video image of the wall with fringe lines resulting from the displacement of the wall by the force exerted by hand.

The second study was a real-time hologram of a graphite/Nomex honeycomb panel located on the wing of a hangared aircraft. The hologram was exposed with a 10 second exposure and reconstructed in real-time. Heat was applied from a heat gun revealing immediately an unbonded area measuring some 4 inches across.

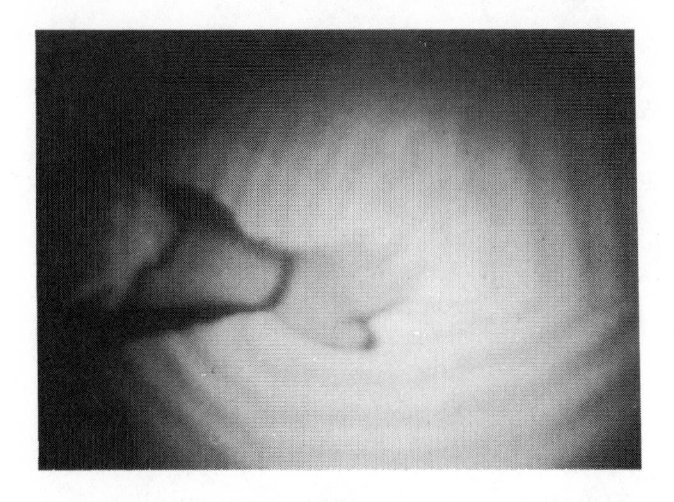

Figure 13. Real-time hologram showing the deformation of a cinderblock wall due to the force from several fingers.

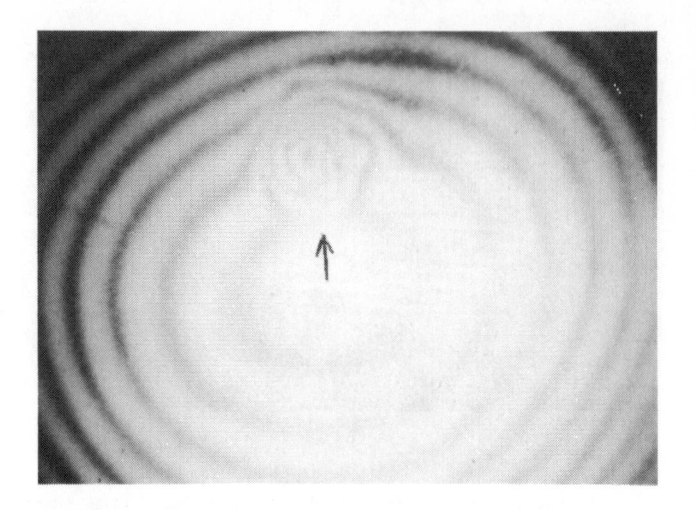

Figure 14. Real-time hologram of a graphite/Nomex honeycomb panel on a hangared aircraft. Arrow points to 4-inch unbond.

Conclusion

In the past three years, holography has grown from a laboratory technique to a powerful tool for industrial nondestructive testing. it is the inspection method of choice in many aircraft applications where it has proven cost benefits. The new techniques of white noise excitation and phase locked holography combined with instant automatic hologram recorders, will place holography in many industrial application not possible until now.

References

1. Erf, R., Holographic Nondestructive Testing, Academic Press, pp. 331. 1974

2. Claraday, J., U.S. Patent 4,408,881
   Issued Oct. 11, 1983

3. Erf, R., Holographic Nondestructive Testing, Academic Press, pp. 306-308. 1974

4. Abramson, N., SPIE Vol. 349, pp. 130. 1982

REVIEW OF PULSED HOLOGRAPHY IN NONDESTRUCTIVE TESTING

Ralph Page
Apollo Lasers, Inc., A subsidiary of Patlex Corporation,
20977 Knapp Street, Chatsworth, California 91311
Robert T. Pitlak
Consultant, 1639 Valecroft Avenue,
Westlake Village, California 91361

ABSTRACT

A review of current applications of pulsed holographic interferometry is followed by a discussion of current limitations to widespread use of the technique. Existing work to overcome the limitations is discussed. A potential new source for pulsed NDT is reviewed.

INTRODUCTION

Pulsed lasers have been used for holographic interferometry for almost 20 years. In 1965, R.E. Brooks, et al[1], reported holograms taken with a Q-switched ruby laser. Soon afterward, a host of work was published regarding holographic interferometry using pulsed laser sources. The vast majority of the work was being performed with the pulsed ruby laser, although other sources (excimer, frequency-doubled YAG) have been used to a lesser degree.

Rapid improvements were made in the coherence, amplitude stability, and output energy of the laser sources, the sensitivity of the recording medium, and experimental techniques. Several analytical techniques for evaluation of the interference fringes were developed.[2-7]

By 1970 several researchers all over the world were performing NDT with pulsed lasers. Excitement ran high. It was predicted that this new technique would soon be utilized for a host of industrial applications. It seemed we were poised at the edge of a new era for NDT. Now, some 15 years later we're still poised for the big push. The authors will review below some of the recent developments that make it reasonable to think that holographic interferometry is, in fact, a viable candidate to compete with or complement the traditional NDT methods now in general use.

First, we will review some current interesting examples of pulsed holographic NDT. Then we will review some interesting new developments in fringe interpretation techniques and laser sources that will make these techniques significantly more accessable to the average NDT technologist.

EXAMPLES OF PULSED HOLOGRAPHIC NDT

Figure 1 is two interferograms of helical lamp cavities. The authors used holographic interferometry to study the effectiveness of acoustic baffles inside the pump cavity to reduce the effect of an acoustic pressure wave created when the lamp fires. Figure 1a is a pump chamber without baffles. Figure 1b is the same pump chamber, equipped with sintered metal acoustic baffles. In both cases, one exposure was taken just as the lamp was fired, and a second was taken 300 microseconds later. The fringes represent expansion of the cover. The lower fringe density in Figure 1b clearly illustrates the effect of the baffles.

Figure 2 shows two holograms taken of an operating engine.[9] This is a good example where a quick, qualitative evaluation of the interferometric fringes can produce meaningful results.

Modern fuel-efficient engines operate at high compression ratios to maximize efficiency. These engines operate on the verge of knocking, and rely on knock sensors to retard the timing just enough to operate smoothly. A small accelerometer is placed on the engine block to act as the knock sensor. The placement of the sensor is critical to optimize signal to noise ratio from the sensor.

A double pulse interferogram was taken of the engine, timed with ignition of one of the cylinders. The pulse separation was fairly short, about 50 microseconds. This minimizes sensitivity to the other low frequency events typical of normal operation.

A second double pulse interferogram was taken of the same engine at the same relative phase, while the engine was knocking. The region of concentric fringes indicated by the arrow shows an obvious area of surface deformation when the engine is knocking. These fringes pinpoint the optimum location for the sensor. This work was done by K. Wanders, H. Weigand, J. Muller, and H. Steinbichler in Koln, West Germany.

Figure 3 is an interferogram of a door on a winter cab kit for the M151 jeep[10]. This is a sheetmetal cab structure that is bolted onto a jeep for winter use. A series of holograms of the door region of the cab were taken while the engine was running at 3,000 RPM. The double pulse laser (300 microsec pulse sep.) was triggered at varying time delays after the #4 spark plug fired. This series of holograms gives an idea of the vibration activity in the door region under operating conditions. This information tells the experimenters what regions of the door are likely to contribute to noise emissions from the structure and can suggest the appropriate location of stiffening ribs to eliminate any substantial displacements. Reducing the noise emitted by a structure with minimum additional cost and weight is naturally a goal for designers. This work was performed at U.S. ARMY Tank-Automotive Command Research and Development Center in Warren, Michigan by Grant Gerhart, Gregory Arutunian and James Graziano.

Figure 4 shows an experimental set-up used by Jim McBain and Bill Stange at Wright Patterson AFB in Ohio to study vibrational modes in rotating structures.[11] A triple pulse ruby laser was used to look at vibrational modes on the rotating bladed disk and determine if the mode was stationary on the disk. A series of three exposures were taken sequentially, to determine if the mode was moving on the disk. The configuration shown in Figure 4 illustrates a method of using the first two pulses of a three pulse train to produce one double pulse hologram and using the second and third pulses to produce a second hologram immediately afterward.

Beamsplitter BS splits off two separate reference beams that are applied to the film from opposite sides of the object. A Pockels cell and reference polarizer in each reference beam path form an electro-optical switch so that only two of the three laser pulses will be transmitted to the hologram. The polarizer is oriented normal to the laser polarization and /2 voltage is applied to the cell to pass a laser pulse. The /2 plate located after the polarizer rotates the light 90° so it is once again vertically polarized for optimum hologram brightness. The rotating disk is viewed through a derotater so the image of the disk is stationary on the film during the exposures.

Figure 5 is the pair of double pulse interferograms produced with the setup in Figure 4. B was taken 250 microsec. after A. You can see the location of the mode on the rotating disk has changed. By measuring the angular difference, and knowing the time difference between interferograms, the rotation rate of the mode can be estimated.

The preceeding examples were only meant to be a representative sample of recent work in pulsed holography for NDT that is being performed now. It, by no means, is a complete review, but the authors feel it is typical of the bulk of the work being done currently.

LASER DEVELOPMENTS

As the examples illustrate, pulsed holographic NDT is still in the development stage. The technique has not found its way into the industrial setting. It has not found the broad usage that was predicated nearly 20 years ago. We will outline the reasons, in the opinions of the authors, the technique has not found broad usage and review how the problems in these areas are being solved.

Pulsed holographic interferometry is a tedious technique that requires a knowledge of optics and the ability to operate a pulsed ruby laser. There are commercially available holocameras that integrate a pulsed ruby laser into an optical configuration that is useful for taking double exposure interferograms. The holocamera simplifies the optical alignment requirements to the degree that a typical technician can maintain the optical alignment of the holocamera optics. This leaves, however, the task of operating the pulsed laser. Commercial lasers are now sufficiently reliable to allow consistant operation with output that has good amplitude stability and long coherence. A pulsed ruby laser, however, has several parameters that must be adjusted properly to provide this stable high quality output. Energy delivered to the lamp, lamp firing timing, electro-optical switch (Q-switch) voltage and timing as well as timing and voltage to any amplifiers that may be used all must be adjusted properly to ensure repeatable stable output. Many ruby laser users find that instead of analyzing data from interferograms, they must spend their time reading laser manuals to assist themselves in producing the desired laser output in the first place.

To be widely accepted, pulsed holographic interferometry must be performed with an easily operated laser source so that obtaining the holograms is not a project in itself.

Apollo Lasers is developing a pulsed ruby laser that should eliminate much of the difficulty in operation of the laser. The power supply for the laser includes an on-board computer. The on-board microcomputer controls the power supply directly and communicates through an RS-232 serial interface to a "host" PC. The host PC allows control of the laser in a simple "user friendly" format and uses algorithms to define all the necessary parameter settings. The user merely requests the desired output energy and pulse separation instead of manually setting all the parameters.

FRINGE INTERPRETATION TECHNIQUES

More important than the ease of use of the laser sources is the issue of data interpretation. Excluding a few cases, the interferometric fringe pattern produced is too complex for intuitive interpretation. Manual analysis is painfully slow and requires a good understanding of the principles of holographic interferometry. Most NDT investigators would prefer not to also become holographic interferometry experts as well. When faced with an interferogram covered with seemingly random fringe patterns, the experimenter can be heard to say, "Where did you put those stain gauges?", or "how much was that finite element software package again?"

An automated, or at least partially automated, analysis system is essential to widespread use of interferometry. Several groups are working on such techniques. The authors will briefly review a couple of approaches.

Y. Katzir[12] et al at the Weizmann Institute in Israel have developed a system shown in Figure 6 for automatic fringe interpretation. The system basically involves fringe counting along one axis. They have done all their work with a CW laser, but the approach can be applied to pulsed work as well.

An interferogram of the object is formed on thermoplastic film and the virtual image of the object is imaged on a linear photodiode array. The object is re-illuminated, and the intensity of the image is stored. Next, the hologram of the object including interferometric fringes is recorded. The first pattern is subtracted from the second (object - object and fringes) to minimize the effect of illumination irregularities. The resultant fringe pattern (along one axis) is smoothed to eliminate noise. Displacements as a function of position can then be computed. A simple cantilevered bar with known flaws was successfully analyzed with this system.

This approach has several limitations. It can be used to observe displacements along one axis only. In the example, a known force was applied, providing an increasing fringe order along the axis of the photodiode arrangement. If the fringe order were not known, or the object was undergoing a complex deformation due to many forcing functions, the fringe order would be nearly impossible to keep track of. Clearly, a more generalized full field approach will be required for general use. Most of the above mentioned limitations were dealt with by Katzir[13] et al with the addition of a "carrier fringe" technique. A major difficulty in automatic fringe analysis is dealing with closed-loop fringes. They are harder for the image processing software to deal with, and it is not possible to determine if the fringe order is increasing or decreasing within the closed-loop set of fringes. To eliminate this problem, a tilt or bias is introduced between exposures of a double exposure interferogram. The result is a set of bias fringes in a predetermined direction through the hologram. The tilt accomplishes two things: All fringes are straight or curved lines. Closed loops have been eliminated, and the relative fringe order throughout the hologram can be determined.

Gilbert et al[14] reported a full field extension of the earlier work by Katzir. A centrally-loaded disk was automatically analyzed, producing a two-dimensional map of deflection. Rather than a linear photodiode array, they used a high resolution vidicon and digitized the entire field.

The state of the art in automatic fringe interpretation is now quite close to being useful for application to general usage on arbitrary objects. All the work the authors are familiar with so far has been done on more idealized structures (cantilevered bars, centrally-loaded disks, etc.), but it looks like we are close to seeing a technique that can handle arbitrary shapes with their accompanying shadows, holes, etc. Hung[15] has indicated that his group is close to completing a technique that will use the bias fringe approach to evaluate arbitrary surfaces.

POTENTIAL NEW LASER SOURCE

With the availability of an easily-operated, reliable pulsed laser, and an automated fringe analysis system for arbitrary objects, pulsed holographic techniques should begin to see much wider usage and acceptance. It is indeed a powerful method of analysis that can be applied to a wide variety of applications.

POTENTIAL NEW LASER SOURCE

The last topic to be covered is discussion of a potential solid state laser source for pulsed holography. With a few rare exceptions, all work in pulsed holography has been performed with ruby lasers or frequency-doubled Nd:YAG lasers. The frequency-doubled YAG lasers can be operated at rep rates of 30HZ or more, but it is difficult to maintain single-mode operation needed for long coherence, and the frequency-doublers only have a typical efficiency of 30% - 40%. As a result, only a fraction of a Joule can be produced at 532 nm.

Alexandrite is a laser material that can overcome some of the limitations inherent in the Nd:YAG laser. Alexandrite has a tunable output that ranges from 720 to 780 nm, and it can be operated at rep rates typical of YAG. The main disadvantage of alexandrite is its wavelength in the near infrared. Agfa-Geavert 10E75 film, which is red-sensitive and designed for HeNe and ruby lasers, begins to lose sensitivity beyond 700 nm.

To evaluate the viability of alexandrite as a source for high rep-rate holography, a standard commercial, multimode alexandrite laser (Apollo Lasers Model 7511) was modified by the authors by adding longitudinal and transverse mode selectors. Several holograms were then taken on Agfa-Geavert 10E75 plates at a wavelength of 725 nm and an output energy of approximately 10 mJ per pulse. We estimated the sensitivity of the film dropped by about 50% at that wavelength, but there was adequate sensitivity to make the hologram shown in Figure 6. Objects about 1 meter behind the statue were clearly visible, indicating a coherence of 2 meters or more. Since the output of the laser can be used without harmonic generators (required with YAG), it is straightforward to increase the laser output with amplifiers. It appears that alexandrite is an excellent candidate as a source of high rep rate, high energy output that could be used for holographic interferometry.

1. R.E. Brooks, L. O. Heflinger, R. F. Wuerker, and R. A. Briones "Holographic Photography of High Speed Phenomena with Conventional and Q-switched Ruby Lasers," Applied Physics Letters, vol. 7, pp. 92-94, August 1965.
2. B. P. Hildebrand and K. A. Haines, Applied Optics 5 (1966) pp. 172-173.
3. K. A. Haines and B. P. Hildebrand, ibid 5 (1966) pp. 595-602.
4. Idem, IEEE Trans. Inst. Meas. 15 (1966) pp. 149-161.
5. E. B. Aleksandrov and A. M. Bonmch-Bruevich, Zh. Tekh. Fiz. 37, (1967) pp. 360-369. (Translation in Sov. Phys. Tech. Phys. 12 (1967) pp. 258-265.)
6. A. E. Ennos, J. Phys. E., J. Sci. Instrum. 1 (1968) pp. 731-734.
7. J. E. Sollid, Applied Optics 8 (1969) pp. 1587-1595.
8. An excellent review of the various interpretation techniques was written by: J. D. Briers, Opt. and Q. Elect. 8 (1976) pp. 469-501.
9. K. Wanders, H. Weigand, J. Muller, H. Steinbichler, "High-Speed Photography and Pulsed Laser Holography for Diagnostic Investigations of Mixture Formation and Vibration in Reciprocating Engines," I. Mechanical Engineering, pp. 79-83.
10. G. Gerhart, G. Arutunian, J. Graziano, U. S. Army Tank-Automotive Command R&D Center Laboratory Tech. Report, No. TR12595, July 1982.
11. J.C. MacBain, W.A. Stange, K.G. Harding, "Analysis of Rotating Structures Using Image Derotation with Multiple Pulsed Lasers and Moire Techniques," SESA Spring Meeting, June 1981, Detroit, Michigan.
12. Y. Katzir, I. Glassman, A. A. Friesem, B. Sharon, "On-Line Acquisition and Analysis for Holographic Evaluation," Optical Engineering, Vol. 21 No. 6, (1966) pp. 1016-1021.
13. Y. Katzir, A. A. Friesem, I. Glasser, B. Sharon, "Holographic Nondestructive Evaluation with Ongoing Acquisition and Processing, Industrial and Commercial Applications of Holography," Milton Chang, Ed. Proceedings of the SPIE 353 (1982) pp. 74-81.
14. J. A. Gilbert, T. D. Dudderar, D. R. Mathys, J. M. Chern, "Digitization of Holographic Interferograms for Deflection Measurement," Proceedings of the 1985 SEM Spring Conference on Experimental Mechanics, June 1985, Las Vegas, Nevada pp. 94-301.
15. M. Hung, Oakland University, Private Communication

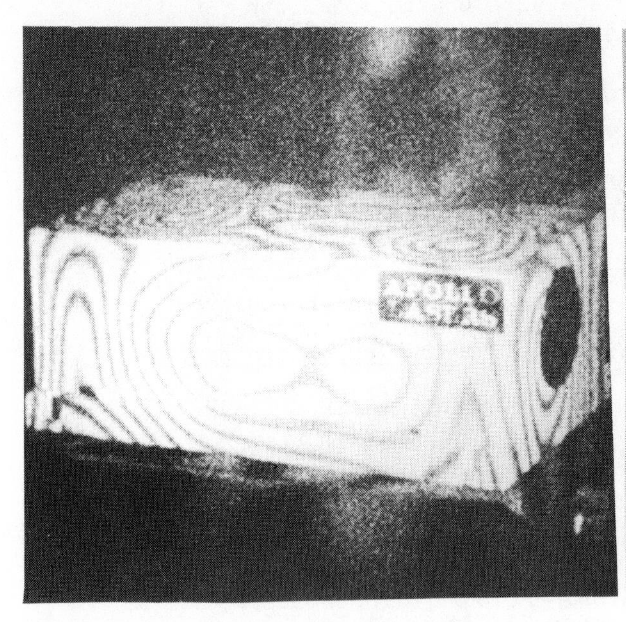

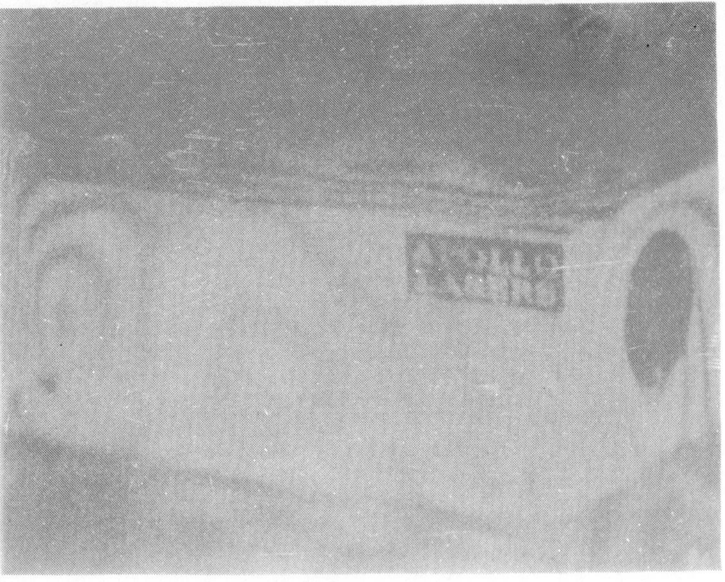

FIGURE 1
LASER HEAD ON LEFT DOES NOT HAVE ACOUSTIC BAFFLES

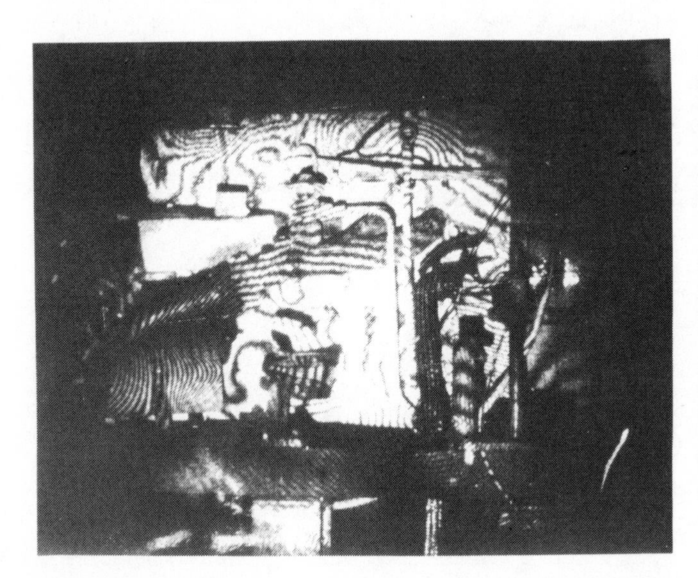

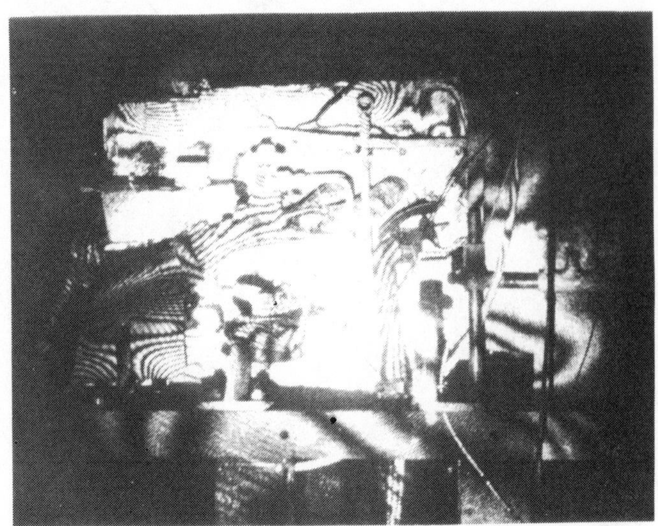

FIGURE 2
OPERATING ENGINE, INTERFEROGRAM ON RIGHT IS KNOCKING
PHOTO COURTESY OF DR. HANS STEINBICHLER

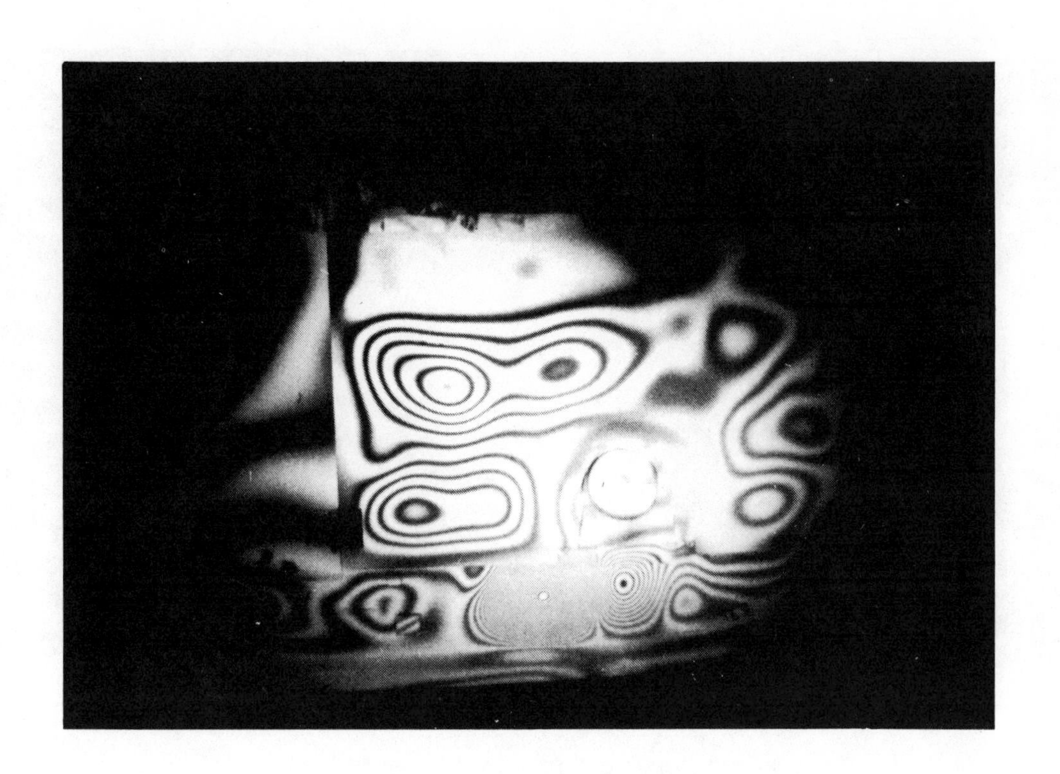

FIGURE 3
WINTER CAB FOR M151 JEEP
PHOTO COURTESY OF GRANT GERHART

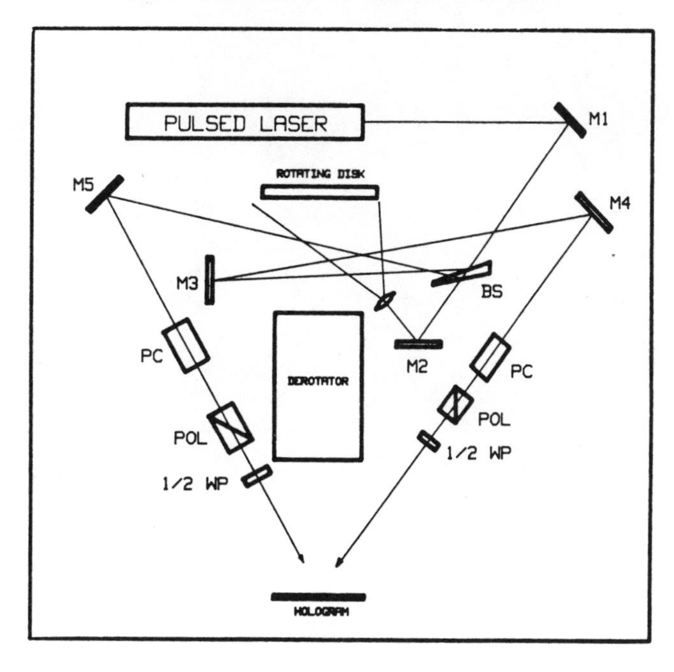

FIGURE 4
OPTICAL CONFIGURATION FOR 3-PULSE HOLOGRAMS

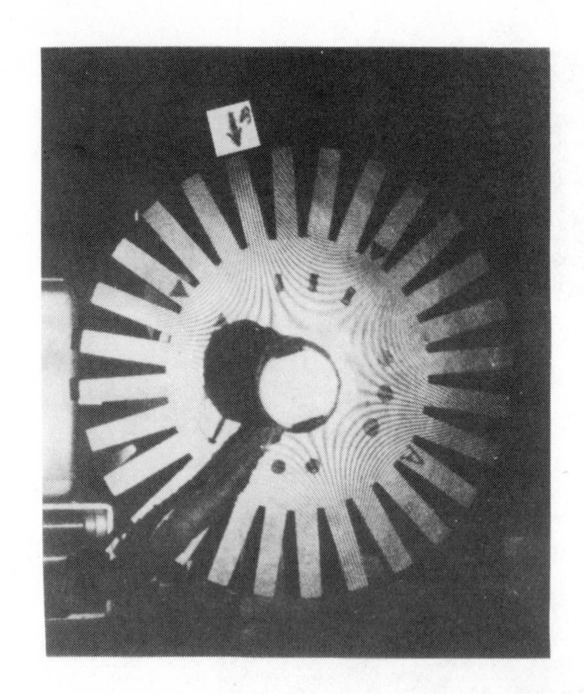

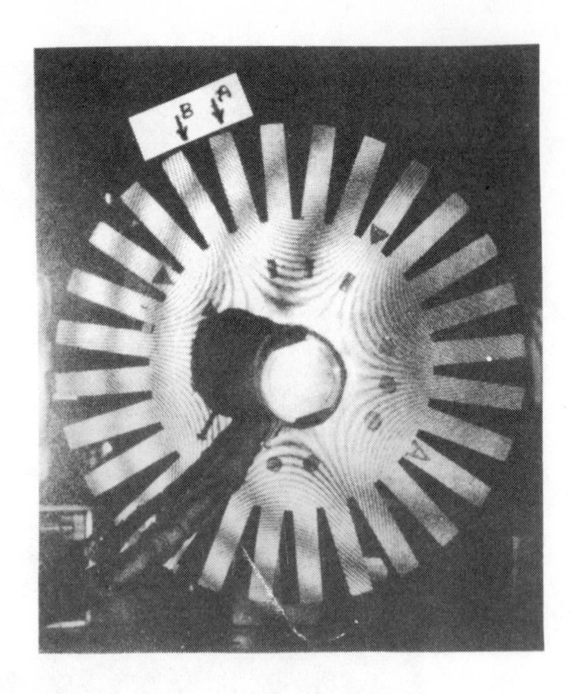

FIGURE 5
ROTATING BLADED DISK
PHOTO COURTESY OF JIM MAC BAIN

FIGURE 6
HOLOGRAM TAKEN WITH ALEXANDRITE LASER

QUANTITATIVE HOLOGRAPHIC ANALYSIS OF SMALL COMPONENTS

Ryszard J. Pryputniewicz

Center for Holographic Studies and Laser Technology
Department of Mechanical Engineering
Worcester Polytechnic Institute, Worcester, Massachusetts 01609

Abstract

Methods of hologram interferometry are used to study load-deflection characteristics of small components. More specifically, fundamentals of the methods of double-exposure hologram interferometry, time average hologram interferometry, and heterodyne hologram interometry are discussed, procedures for quantitative interpretation of holograms are outlined, and their applications are illustrated by representative examples. Results presented in this paper indicate viability of the methods of hologram interferometry for quantitative studies of small components.

Introduction

Today's demands for optimum design of small components, in particular in respect to electronic packaging, require accurate knowledge of the behavior of components under actual operating conditions. This information, however, is difficult to obtain experimentally because of the small size of the today's components. Also, the conventional experimental procedures, involving strain gauges, photoelasticity, mechanical probing, etc., are generally not applicable to these measurements because they are invasive in nature and, therefore, interfere with the performance of the tested component. An alternative to the conventional experimental methods, however, can be provided using recent developments in laser methods.

Out of a number of the existing laser methods, available today, hologram interferometry was found to be most applicable to the studies of small components, as presented in this paper. This stems from the fact that displacements and/or deformations of the components are very small and take place over the entire component, which itself is very small, on the order of a few millimeters in physical dimensions. Also, methods used to make measurements, on such components, must assure accurate and precise results. Otherwise, experimental uncertainties will constitute an appreciable percentage of the measured quantity and the experimental results might not be useful from the designer's point of view.

The results presented in this paper were obtained using the methods of double-exposure hologram interferometry, time average hologram interferometry, and heterodyne hologram interferometry to study displacements and strains of small components. The following sections detail the methods used, the laboratory apparatus employed in the study, and the results obtained.

Methods used

In the study presented in this paper, the methods of double-exposure hologram interferometry, time average hologram interferometry, and heterodyne hologram interferometry were used, as detailed below.

Double-exposure hologram interferometry

Out of the variety of the existing holographic procedures, the most suitable for studies of small components is the double-exposure method. In this method, two consecutive positions of an object are recorded in the same recording medium, with the object being displaced and deformed between the two exposures.[1] Upon reconstruction of the hologram, two three-dimensional images of the object are formed. Since both images appear in coherent (laser) light and exist in approximately the same location in space, they interfere with each other and produce fringes "covering" the reconstructed image. All information about the object's motion and deformation can be determined from this fringe pattern.

A typical setup for recording and reconstruction of double-exposure holograms is shown in Fig. 1. In this setup, the highly coherent and monochromatic light from a laser is divided into two parts by means of a beamsplitter. One of these parts, going straight through the beamsplitter, is directed by a mirror and expanded by a lens to illuminate an object to be recorded. This part of the laser output is known as the <u>object beam</u>. The other part of the laser beam, that is, the one which is reflected from the beam splitter, is expanded and

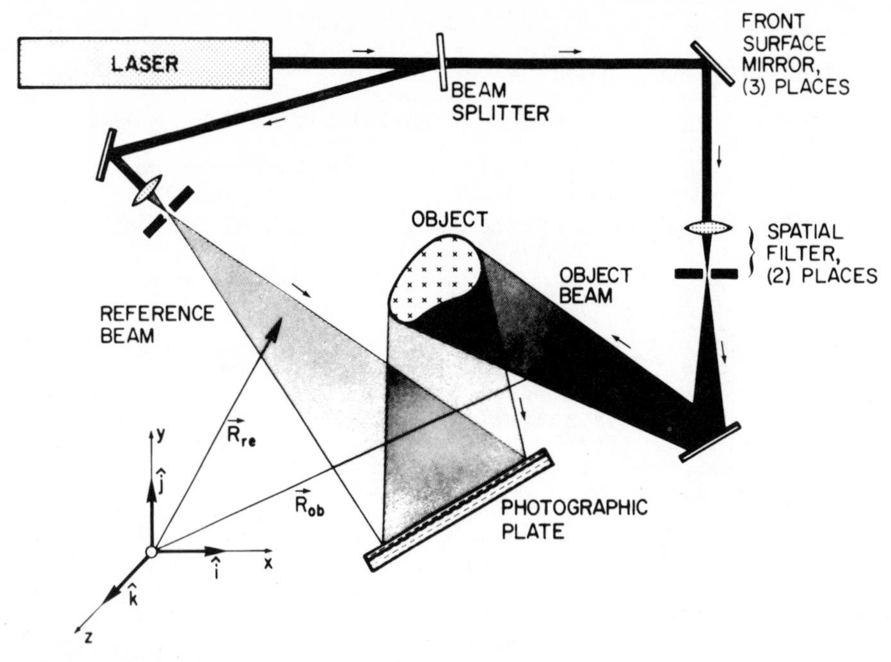

Fig. 1. A setup for recording and reconstruction of double-exposure holograms: x, y, and z represent axes of the rectangular coordinate system, with $\hat{i}$, $\hat{j}$, and $\hat{k}$ being corresponding unit vectors, while $\underline{\underline{R}}_{ob}$ and $\underline{\underline{R}}_{re}$ are position vectors defining the object and the reference beams, respectively.

steered toward a high resolution medium without any interference with the object. This beam provides a reference beam against which the light modulated by the object is "compared" when they are combined at the photographic medium. The superposition of the object and the reference beams results in an interference pattern which is recorded by the high resolution recording medium. The exposed high resolution medium, upon processing, becomes a hologram. The hologram can be used to reconstruct the three-dimensional image of the original object. During this process, the hologram is, most conveniently, illuminated with the original reference beam. The image produced, during reconstruction of the hologram, is seen covered with a fringe pattern which uniquely relates to motions and/or deformations that the object experienced during recording of the hologram[2]. Some of the procedures for quantitative interpretation of holograms are outlined in this paper.

Time average hologram interferometry

Time average holograms can be recorded using a setup similar to that shown in Fig. 2. In time average hologram interferometry, a single holographic recording of an object, undergoing a cyclic vibration, is made. With the (continuous) exposure time long in comparison to one period of the vibration cycle, the hologram effectively records an ensemble of images corresponding to the time average of all positions of the object while it is vibrating. During reconstruction of such a hologram, the interference occurs between the entire ensemble of images, with the image recorded near zero velocity (that is, maximum displacement) contributing most strongly to the reconstruction. The interference fringes observed are of unequal brightness. In fact, they vary according to the square of the zero-order Bessel function of the first kind[3-5] that is, J_0^2. The J_0 fringes, observed during reconstruction of time average holograms, differ from cosinusoidal fringes obtained in double-exposure hologram interferometry. One of these differences is that the zero-order J_0 fringe represents the stationary points on the vibrating object and thus allows easy identification of nodes. The brightness of other J_0 fringes, as well as their spacing, decrease with increasing fringe order and can be directly related to mode shapes.

The time average hologram interferometry is the most popular of the holographic methods for vibration analysis. The existing holographic laboratories are, in general well equipped to perform time average studies. The apparatus is the same as that used in recording of conventional holograms, except for the mechanism to "drive" the object. The driving mechanism can be a piezoelectric shaker, a loud speaker, a magnetic oscillator, a flowing fluid, etc. However, regardless of the method used, to excite the object, the time-averaged interference fringes are the same in nature.

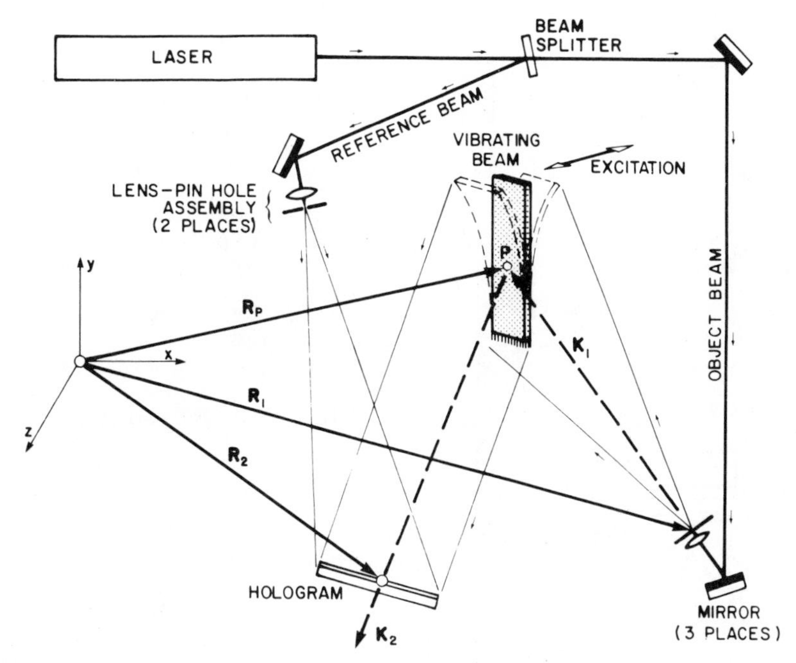

Fig. 2. A setup for recording and reconstruction of time average holograms: $\underline{\underline{R}}_1$, $\underline{\underline{R}}_2$, and $\underline{\underline{R}}_P$ are position vectors defining point-source of illumination, point of observation, and a point on the object, respectively, while $\underline{\underline{K}}_1$ and $\underline{\underline{K}}_2$ represent directions of object illumination and observation, respectively.

Heterodyne hologram interferometry

The characteristic principle of heterodyne hologram interferometry is that each of the two object fields (in the case of the double-exposure method) is recorded with a different reference beam[6]. These recordings are made in the high resolution photosensitive medium. The reference beams are set up in such a way that they can be reproduced independently, during the hologram reconstruction process, with an introduction of a known frequency shift between them. As a result of this, the two reconstructed and interfering light fields are intensity modulated at the frequency equal to the frequency shift between the reference beams. This intensity modulation takes place at all points within the interference pattern produced during reconstruction of the hologram. The optical path differences, corresponding to the displacement and/or deformation recorded within the hologram being reconstructed, are converted into phase of the beat frequency of the two interfering light fields. This phase is, in turn, interpolated opto-electronically, resulting in highly accurate determination of displacements and/or strains.

Recording and reconstruction of heterodyne holograms can be made using a system similar to that shown in Fig. 3. In this arrangement, laser output is divided into three beams by means of beamsplitters BS1 and BS2. The first beam, reflected from BS1, is directed by mirror M1, via beam expander BE1, toward the recording medium H; this is the reference beam R1. The second beam, reflected from BS2, is the reference beam R2. The third beam, directed by mirrors M3 and M4, is expanded by BE3 to illuminate the object being studied. This beam, modulated by reflection from the object, is recorded against R1 and R2, one at a time, with the exposure being controlled by shutters S1 and S2, respectively, as described below.

Using the heterodyne holography arrangement shown in Fig. 3, the object's configuration C1, corresponding to its initial state, is recorded using the object beam and R1 while R2 is stopped by S2. Following the first exposure, state of the object is altered resulting in configuration C2. Then, the second exposure is made, in the same photographic medium, recording C2. This second recording, however, is made using the object beam and R2, while R1 is blocked by S1. It should be noted that during the two exposures, the object beam as well as R1 and R2 all have the same frequency.

The exposed photosensitive medium is processed and then reconstructed by simultaneous illumination with R1 and R2, while the object beam is stopped by S3. Now, however, a frequency shift is introduced between R1 and R2 be means of the acousto-optic modulators AM1 and AM2, which are cascaded in R2. Therefore, the two light fields A_1 and A_2, corresponding to the reference beams R1 and R2, respectively, can be expressed as functions of position vectors $\underline{\underline{R}}$ and time τ, that is,

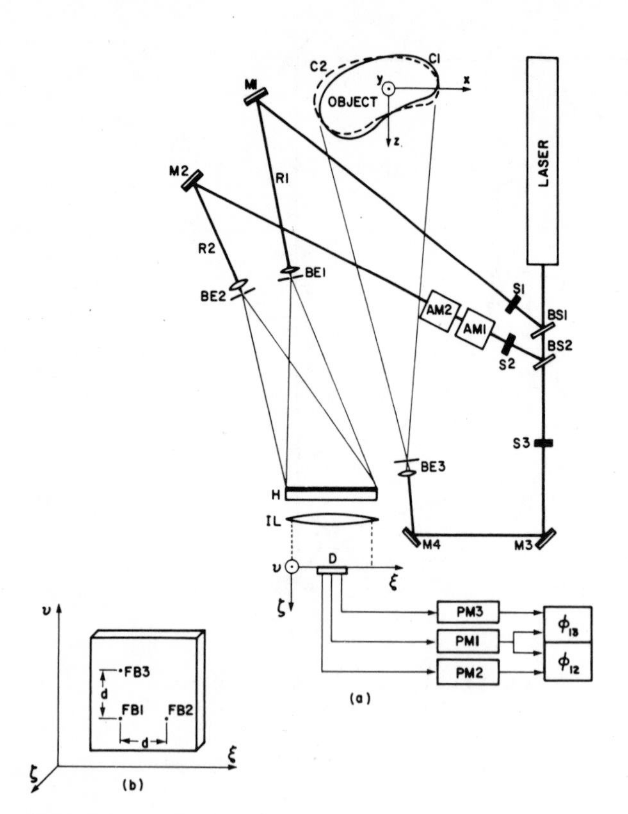

Fig. 3. Heterodyne system: a) system setup - BS1 and BS2 are beamsplitters, S1 to S3 are shutters, M1 to M4 are mirrors, AM1 and AM2 are acousto-optic modulators, BE1 to BE3 are beam expanders, R1 and R2 are reference beams, H is a hologram, D is a detector, PM1 to PM3 are phase meters; b) fiber-optic detector head - FB1 to FB3 are fiber-optic bundles, d is the center-to-center distance between the fiber-optic bundle pairs.

$$A_1(\mathbf{R},\tau) = a_1(\mathbf{R}) \exp i\left[\omega_1\tau + \phi_1(\mathbf{R})\right] , \tag{1}$$

and

$$A_2(\mathbf{R},\tau) = a_2(\mathbf{R}) \exp i\left[\omega_2\tau + \phi_2(\mathbf{R})\right] , \tag{2}$$

where a represents real amplitudes, ω represents frequencies, ϕ represents phases, and subscripts 1 and 2 denote reconstructing beams R1 and R2, respectively. A photodetector D, Fig. 3a, placed at a point within the image formed by an imaging lens IL, detects intensity variation, $I(\underline{\underline{R}},t)$, in any region of space where the two light fields overlap, that is,

$$I(\mathbf{R},\tau) = a_1^2(\mathbf{R}) + a_2^2(\mathbf{R}) + 2a_1(\mathbf{R})a_2(\mathbf{R}) \cos\left[\omega_{12}\tau + \phi_{12}(\mathbf{R})\right] , \tag{3}$$

where

$$\phi_{12}(\mathbf{R}) = \phi_2(\mathbf{R}) - \phi_1(\mathbf{R}) \tag{4}$$

is the interference phase (that is, optical phase difference between the two light fields) appearing as the phase of the intensity modulation at the beat frequency ω_{12}. This beat frequency equals to the frequency difference between the two reconstructing beams, viz.,

$$\omega_{12} = \omega_2 - \omega_1 . \tag{5}$$

In the setup used to obtain results presented in this paper, a detector assembly consisting of three fiber-optic bundles FB1, FB2, and FB3, Fig. 3b, was used. The signals from the fiber-optic bundles were fed into photomultipliers PM1, PM2, and PM3, respectively. The outputs from the photomultipliers were, in turn, sensed and displayed by the differential phasemeters, as shown in Fig. 3a. The phase differences, measured at a number of points in the image formed by IL, were then automatically fed into a dedicated computer which performed all of the computations to determine displacements and strains of small components.

In deformation analysis, the first and the second derivatives, $\underline{\underline{L}}'$ and $\underline{\underline{L}}''$, respectively, of the displacement vector $\underline{\underline{L}}$ are calculated. In general, for the nth point, these derivatives can be approximated numerically as

$$L'_{i_n} = \frac{L_{i_{n+1}} - L_{i_{n-1}}}{d} , \tag{6}$$

and

$$L''_{i_n} = \frac{L_{i_{n+2}} - 2L_{i_n} + L_{i_{n-2}}}{d^2} , \tag{7}$$

where i denotes axes of the rectangular coordinate system, $L_{i_{n-2}}$, $L_{i_{n-1}}$, L_{i_n}, etc., represent displacement components of points n-2, n-1, n, etc., which are separated by the distance d/2. If the distance d, appearing in Eqs 6 and 7 is equal to the separation of two fiber-optic bundles in the detector head assembly, Fig. 3b, then the first derivatives of the displacement vector $\underline{\underline{L}}_{ob}$, observed in the image plane formed by IL (that is, $\underline{\underline{L}}_{ob} = L_\xi \hat{i} + L_\upsilon \hat{j}$), can be related to the corresponding phase differences as

$$L'_{\xi_n} = \frac{L_{\xi_{n+1}} - L_{\xi_{n-1}}}{d} = \frac{1}{d}\left(\frac{\phi_{n+1}}{2\pi}\lambda - \frac{\phi_{n-1}}{2\pi}\lambda\right) = \frac{\lambda}{2\pi d}\left(\phi_2 - \phi_1\right) = \frac{\lambda}{2\pi d}\phi_{12} , \tag{8}$$

and

$$L'_{\nu_n} = \frac{\lambda}{2\pi d}\phi_{13} \quad , \tag{9}$$

where λ is the wavelength of laser light used in recording and reconstruction of the hologram. The ϕ_{12}, appearing in Eq. 8, is the phase difference between the signals detected by fiber-optic bundles FB1 and FB2 arranged parallel to the ξ-axis, Fig. 3b, while ϕ_{13} (see Eq. 9) corresponds to the signals sensed by FB1 and FB3, arranged parallel to the ν-axis. In a similar manner, the second derivatives of displacement, Eq. 7, can also be represented in terms of the measured local phase differences[6].

Quantitative interpretation of holograms

In applications of hologram interferometry to studies of small components, it is often desired to investigate objects for which the entire surface has moved and/or deformed. In such applications, it is not possible to determine true fringe orders and, therefore, conventional procedures of hologram interpretation do not apply, because these procedures are based on indentification of the zero-order fringe. In fact, mathematical procedures for interpretation of fringe patterns where the zero-order fringe is present are simpler than those where the zero-order fringe is not identifiable. This latter case, however, is what usually takes place during applications of hologram interferometry to studies of small components.

Determination of displacements

To obtain quantitative results from fringe patterns produced during reconstruction of holograms, parameters characterizing recording and reconstruction geometry must be determined. This geometry is specified by identifying point-source from which object is illuminated, point(s) of interest on the object, and direction(s) of observation along which the reconstructed image is viewed, Fig. 4.

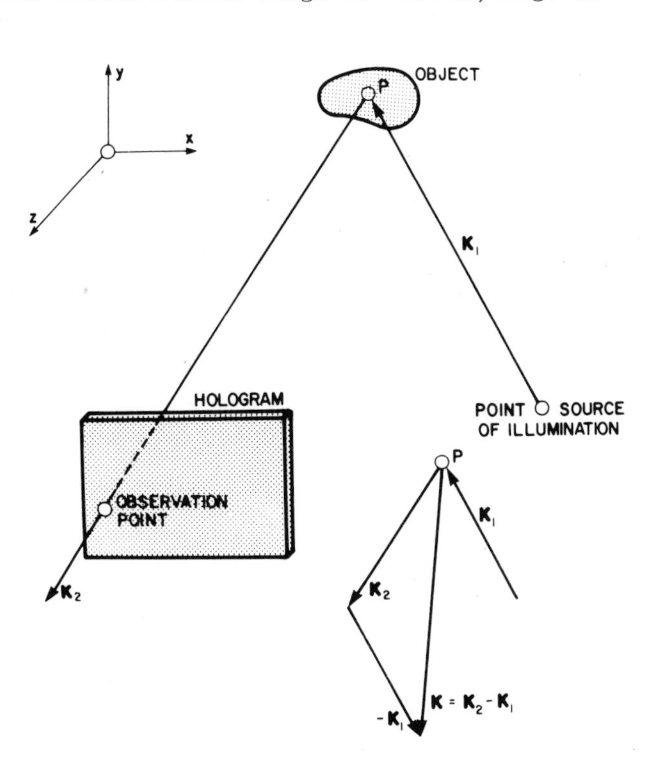

Fig. 4. Illumination and observation geometry for quantitative interpretation of holograms: $\underline{\underline{K}}_1$ is the vector defining direction of object illumination, $\underline{\underline{K}}_2$ is the vector defining direction of observation, $\underline{\underline{K}}$ is the sensitivity vector defined as the difference between $\underline{\underline{K}}_1$ and $\underline{\underline{K}}_2$.

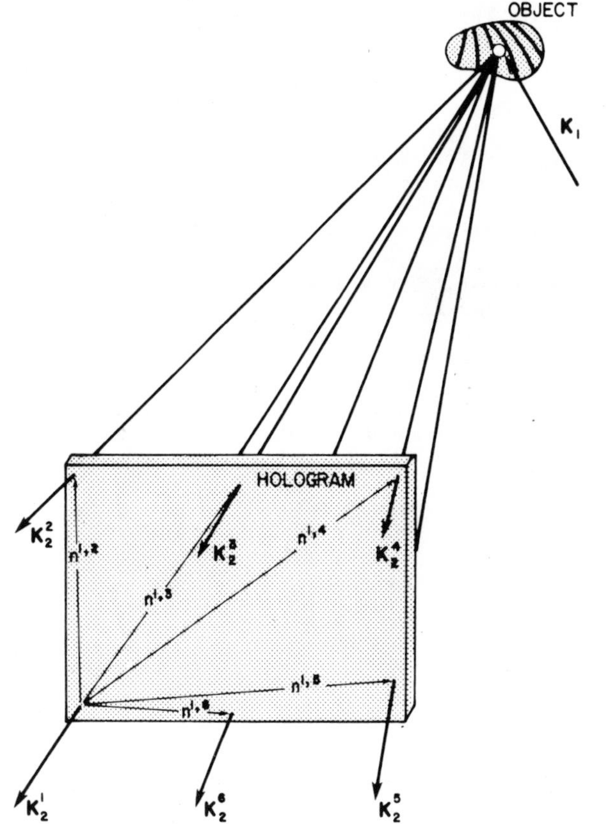

Fig. 5. Multiple observations of holographically reconstructed image: $\underline{\underline{K}}_1$ is the vector defining direction of illumination, $\underline{\underline{K}}_2^1$ to $\underline{\underline{K}}_2^6$ are vectors defining directions of observation, while $n^{1,2}$ to $n^{1,5}$ represent changes in fringe orders observed during the corresponding changes in the directions of observation.

Very commonly, these parameters are determined making only one observation of the holographically reconstructed image, assuming that the motion of the object was in the plane normal to the direction of observation. This approach might generally work in laboratory with inanimate objects where experimenter can carefully control test conditions. However, even in this "static" case, the resulting accuracy of the measurements, obtained from one observation only, is questionable due to errors in determination of various experimental parameters. On the other hand, use of multiple observations of holographically reconstructed images, Fig. 5, leads to accurate and precise determination of object motions.[1]

In applications of hologram interferometry to studies of small components, it is of interest to measure motions, changes under load, "growth" patterns, etc., which are all three-dimensional in nature and, as such, parameters quantifying them can best be described by vectors. Since vectors are completely defined by specifying their three components, then, working with holography, one is usually dealing with three unknowns. These unknowns are the three components of the vector defining quantity of interest. Using vector calculus, governing equations of hologram interferometry can be written in such a way that one equation will relate one component of the unknown vector to parameters characterizing fringe patterns as determined from one direction of observation.[1] Thus, ideally, three equations, that is, one for each of the three observations, should be sufficient to quantitatively interpret holograms. In theory, the procedure works. In practice, however, the results are often subjected to large uncertainties because of experimental errors in determination of parameters used in computations.[2]

To overcome the above difficulty, a method of interpretation of holograms, based on multiple observations and resulting in an overdetermined system of equations, that is, a system having more equations than the number of unknowns, was developed.[1] It was also shown that as the number of observations increases so does the accuracy of the corresponding results.

In the method of multiple observations of a hologram, the scalar product of the object's vectorial displacement $\underline{\underline{L}}$ with the sensitivity vector $\underline{\underline{K}}$ is related to the fringe order n by the equation

$$\mathbf{K} \cdot \mathbf{L} = 2\pi n = \Omega , \tag{10}$$

where Ω is the fringe-locus function, constant values of which define fringe loci on the surface of the object, while Ω_0 is a constant to be determined from the observed fringe pattern. The sensitivity vector $\underline{\underline{K}}$, appearing in Eq. 10, is defined as a difference between the observation vector $\underline{\underline{K}}_2$ and the illumination vector $\underline{\underline{K}}_1$, Fig. 4, that is,

$$\mathbf{K} = \mathbf{K}_2 - \mathbf{K}_1 \ . \tag{11}$$

In this way, for each observation of the image reconstructed from the hologram, one equation of the type of Eq. 10 can be written, ralating the observation/illumination geometry and the fringe orders to the unknown displacement vector. Generally, four observations are required in order to determine the vectorial motion of the object and the constant Ω_0. However, it is common in holographic analysis to use more than four observations in order to reduce experimental errors.[1] In cases such as this, solution is made for the four parameters that yield the least-square-error, in an attempt to satisfy the overdetermined set of equations that is generated from the excess data.

Using the method of multiple observations, the image reconstructed from the hologram can be viewed as shown in Fig. 5, and the system of simultaneous equations, corresponding to these multiple observations can be solved to obtain the displacement vector $\underline{\underline{L}}$ and the constant Ω_0, that is,

$$\begin{pmatrix} \mathbf{L} \\ \Omega_0 \end{pmatrix} = \left[\underset{\sim}{G}^T \underset{\sim}{G} \right]^{-1} \left(\underset{\sim}{G}^T \Delta \Omega \right) , \tag{12}$$

where Ω_0 is equivalent to the fringe order that would have been assigned to the fringe passing the point of interest on the object, while observing it along the direction $\underline{\underline{K}}_2^1$ had the zero-order fringe been identifiable; the matrix $\underset{\sim}{G}$ represents the sensitivity vectors corresponding to the multiple observations of the image.

In the case of time average holograms of vibrating components, when excitation causes the principal motion of an object in the direction parallel to the z-axis, Fig. 2, the displacement of the object is[4]

$$L_z = \frac{\lambda}{2\pi\left(\hat{K}_{2_z} - \hat{K}_{1_z}\right)} \left|\Omega_t\right| \quad , \tag{13}$$

where L_z is the displacement of a vibrating object, λ is laser wavelength, Ω_t is the argument of J_0, and $(\hat{K}_{2z} - \hat{K}_{1z})$ represents the sensitivity vector in the direction of displacement.

For the case of retro-reflective illumination and observation, parallel to the z-axis, the quantity $(\hat{K}_{2z} - \hat{K}_{1z})$ has the maximum value of 2 and Eq. 13 reduces to

$$L_z = \frac{\lambda}{4\pi}\left|\Omega_t\right| \quad . \tag{14}$$

However, for any geometry where the directions of illumination and observation are not parallel to the z-axis, the quantity $(\hat{K}_{2z} - \hat{K}_{1z})$ will always be less than 2. Its actual magnitude will depend on the magnitudes of angles that the directions of $\underline{\underline{K}}_1$ and $\underline{\underline{K}}_2$ make with the direction of $\underline{\underline{L}}$. That is, for every case when directions of illumination and observation deviate from being parallel to the directions of motion, the L_z computed from Eq. 13 will always be greater than that given by Eq. 14, for the same order of the J_0 fringe.[7]

The displacements obtained from Eqs 12 to 14 may contain rather complex information relating to desired object motions superposed onto undesired motions such as those due to rigid-body motions[8]. To assure that the measured motions are correct, additional computations determining magnitudes and directions of the unwanted motions must be performed.

Determination of strains and rotations

Currently, there are a number of methods for strain measurement from holograms, including the opto-electronic fringe interpolation method[6,9] the fringe localization method,[10] phase step method,[11] and the fringe vector method.[1,2]

The fringe vector method, used to obtain results presented in this paper, is based on the fact that any combination of homogeneous strain, shear, and rotation of an object yields fringes on its surface which can be described by a single vector. If an object undergoes a deformation and/or rotation, while recording a hologram then, during the reconstruction, the object will be seen covered by a pattern of fringes that would appear to be generated along the lines of intersection of the object's surface with a set of surfaces called fringe-locus surfaces. The fringe-locus surfaces are uniquely defined by the fringe vector whose magnitude is inversely proportional to the spacing between these surfaces and whose direction is normal to them. As such, the fringe vector $\underline{\underline{K}}_f$ can be expressed in terms of the matrix $\tilde{f}$ of strains, shears, and rotations of the object, and the first order variations of the sensitivity vector described by the matrix $\tilde{g}$, that is,

$$\mathbf{K}_f = \mathbf{K}\tilde{f} + \mathbf{L}\tilde{g} \quad . \tag{15}$$

What is of interest in Eq. 15 is the matrix $\tilde{f}$ which can be decomposed into a matrix of strains and shears, $\tilde{e}$, and a matrix of rotations, $\tilde{\theta}$.

In order to solve Eq. 15 for the strain-rotation matrix $\tilde{f}$, multiple observations of the holographically produced image must be made. For each observation the sensitivity vector $\underline{\underline{K}}$ and the fringe vector $\underline{\underline{K}}_f$ must be determined that best fit the data from the entire region examined. Also, multiple views are used to obtain displacement $\underline{\underline{L}}$ at a point of interest on the object. For each view, the matrix $\tilde{g}$ is computed and multiplied by $\underline{\underline{L}}$ to obtain perspective correction to $\underline{\underline{K}}_f$. From multiple views, a set of equations of the type of Eq. 15, with the matrix $\tilde{f}$ common to all equations, is generated and solved to obtain

$$\tilde{f} = \left[\tilde{K}^T \tilde{K}\right]^{-1}\left[\tilde{K}^T \tilde{K}_{fc}\right] \quad , \tag{16}$$

where $\tilde{K}_{f_c} = \tilde{K}_f - \underline{\underline{L}}\tilde{g}$ is the matrix formed by the fringe vectors corrected for perspective. Decomposition of the matrix $\tilde{f}$, computed from Eq. 16, into the symmetric part $\tilde{e}$ and the antisymmetric part $\tilde{\theta}$, that is,

$$\tilde{e} = \frac{1}{2}\left[\tilde{f} + \tilde{f}^T\right] \tag{17}$$

and

$$\tilde{\theta} = \frac{1}{2}\left[\tilde{f} - \tilde{f}^T\right] \quad , \tag{18}$$

gives strains and shears, and rotations, respectively.

Experimental setup

In the study presented in this paper, printed circuit boards were subjected to mechanical, thermal, ans "flow" induced loads.

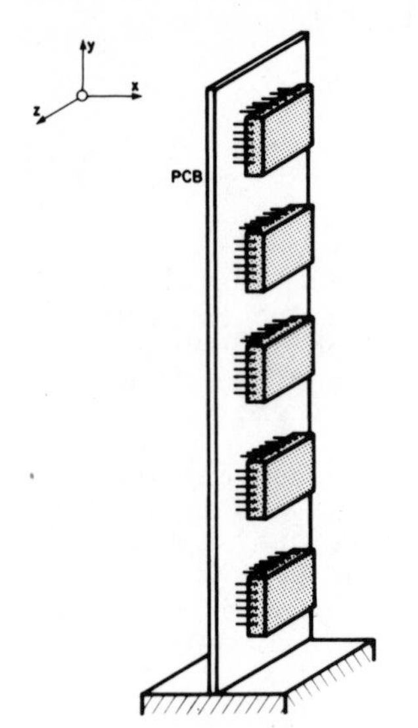

Fig. 6. Configuration of the printed circuit board with surface mounted components.

The board, with surface mounted devices, was assembled as a cantilever plate, Fig. 6, with its upper end free to deflect. Also, a mechanical loading device was attached, in such a way as to provide a known deflection at the free end of the board, at a known frequency.

In addition to the flexural loads, another board was subjected to localized thermal loads. Also, in a different study, boards were subjected to vibrational excitation.

Images of components, produced during reconstruction of holograms, were magnified optically to facilitate their quantitative interpretation. In the case of heterodyne hologram interferometry, local difference measurements were made by moving the fiber-optic detector head (Fig. 3) in the plane of the magnified image of the component. For example, when measuring load-deflection characteristics of the leads the detector was moved along the center of each of the leads by changing its position in increments of 1 mm (as measured in the image space). In this way, it was possible to make measurements at 40 (forty) points along each lead, including the board-lead solder joint and the lead-component centerface.

The data provided by these measurements can be thought of being equivalent to information that could have been obtained if it were possible to place 40 (forty) strain gages along each lead. In fact, the measurements made within the image formed during reconstruction of the heterodyne holograms do relate directly to the components' response to the applied loads.

The phase difference measurements made from the heterodyne holograms were, in turn, used to compute displacements and strains of the tested component, as detailed in the next section.

Experimental results

Results presented in this section are divided into three parts. Part I deals with the calibration data, with particular emphasis on demonstration of the accuracy of the double-exposure heterodyne hologram interferometry as applied to the studies of small components. Part II deals with the studies of the load-deflection characteristics of small components subjected to flexural loads. Part III deals with results showing components' response to thermal and to dynamic loads.

Calibration data

To demonstrate accuracy of the heterodyne hologram interferometry, as applied to the studies of small components, double-exposure holograms were recorded, without any load applied to the board. The image reconstructed from this "no load" double-exposure hologram is shown in Fig. 7. Clearly, during reconstruction of these holograms, no fringes are seen anywhere on the object indicating no "apparent" motion. Therefore, ideally, when the measurements are made from such a hologram, the resulting displacements and strains should be zero. However, due to the optical and electronic noise, some finite phase difference measurements were recorded which, in turn, have resulted in very small displacements and strains, Fig. 8.

Figure 8a shows the component board geometry and the loading condition indicating that, in this case, no load was applied to the board.

Figure 8b shows displacement versus position for Lead-1, under the "no load" condition. Although, for this case, the displacement should ideally be "zero", its actual values range between +/- 0.001 μm, with the average displacement being -0.000,32 μm. Statistical analysis of the 40 point displacement data sample (shown in Fig. 8b) resulted in the standard deviation of 0.000,407 μm, which for the 99.7% confidence interval (that is, for the interval of +/- 3 standard deviations) yielded an uncertainty in the displacement measurement of +/- 0.001,22 μm. In a similar manner, uncertainties in displacement measurements for Lead-2 through Lead-6 were also determined. Examination of these data

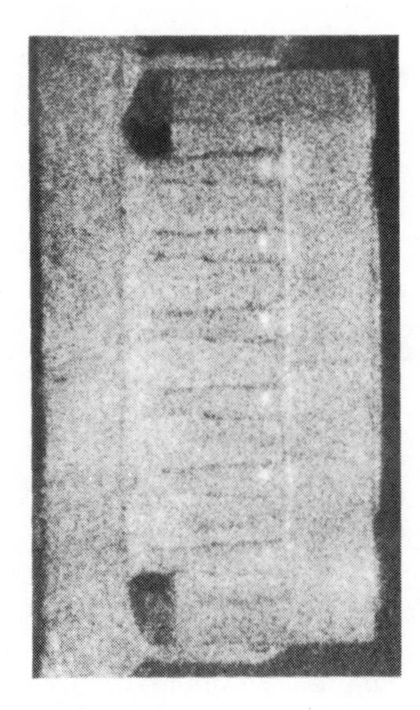

Fig. 7. A typical image produced during reconstruction of a double-exposure heterodyne hologram of a component at no load condition.

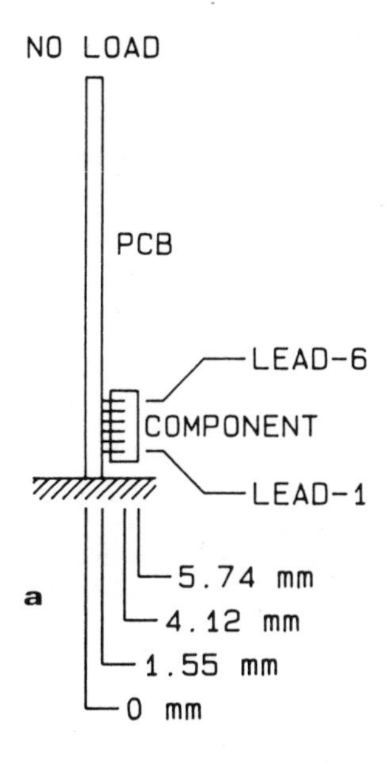

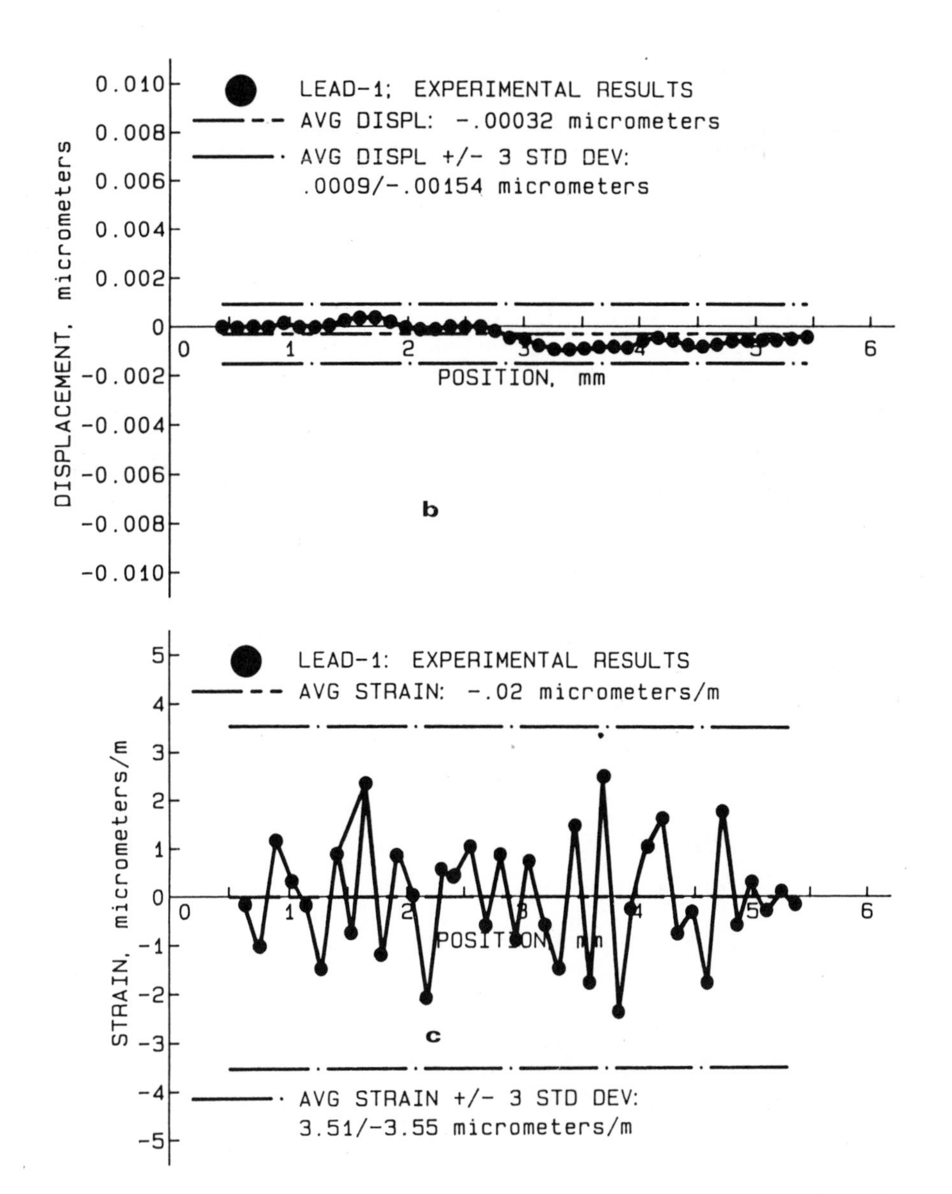

Fig. 8. Calibration data: a) component geometry and loading condition, b) displacement versus position for Lead-1, c) strain versus position for Lead-1.

showed that while using heterodyne hologram interferometry to mesure displacements of the leads, the uncertainty is 0.002 µm, for the 99.7% confidence interval in the displacement measurement.

Figure 8c displays the strain versus position for Lead-1 under the no load condition. Ideally, for this case, the strain readings should be zero. However, the strains measured from the heterodyne holograms indicate values ranging within +/- 0.000,3% (that is, +/- 3 µm/m), with the average strain of -0.000,002%. The statistical analysis of the measured strain yielded the standard deviation of 0.000,117,7%, which for the 99.7% confidence interval resulted in the uncertainty of +/- 0.000,353% in the strain measurement. The bahavior of the strain versus position data characteristics for Lead-2 through Lead-6 was measured to be similar to that for the Lead-1. Based on these results, the overall uncertainty in strain measurement was determined to be 0.000,4%.

Load-deformation data

To determine the load-deformation characteristics of the leads, a series of double-exposure holograms were recorded under different load conditions. A typical image obtained during reconstruction of the corresponding holograms is shown in Fig. 9.

It should be noted that similar - in appearance - fringe patterns were obtained for both positive and negative loads, the only difference was the sign of the corresponding displacement vector which was reflected in the sign of the measured phase differences. The holograms were recorded while board flexing was stopped at a desired position on the sinusoidal loading cycle. Ideally, these holograms should have been recorded under denamic loading conditions. However, to do this, a pulsed laser would be needed and one was not available for this study. Therefore, recordings of all holograms were made using a CW Ar-ion laser while the board was stationary during the exposures.

To obtain data on load-deformation of the component board assembly, holograms were recorded for various magnitudes of deflection. Representative results, corresponding to these holograms, are shown in Fig. 10.

For this representative case, Fig. 10a displays a schematic diagram of the board assembly showing the test component and the loading condition. Shown in this figure are also pertinent dimensions indicating locations necessary to establish positions of the board-lead solder joint and the lead-component interface. Figures 10b and 10c, on the other hand, give the summary of the displacement versus position results and strain versus position results, respectively. The summary figures are useful in determining the displacement/strain trends under given conditions of the test.

Results of this study indicate that although there is a minimal displacement at the board-lead solder joint, there is a considerable non-zero displacement at the lead-component interface. In general, the outermost leads (that is, Lead-1 and Lead-6) show lower overall displacement than the inner four leads. The maximum displacement at any point on the leads does not exceed 1.2 µm. It should also be noted that reversing the direction of the load at the board's tip, causes also a reverse in the leads' displacement direction. For the cases when the load was positive and resulted in the leads pushing against the component, the leads "buckled" outward, that is, away from the component. However, application of the negative load, which "pulled" the component, caused the leads to "move" inward, that is, toward the component.

The data on strain distribution indicate that there are "rapid" changes in strain levels and directions at the points corresponding to the board-lead solder joint and the lead-component interface, respectively. However, the strain distributions along the leads vary approximately linearly. From these data it is seen that strains up to 540 µm/m (or 0.054%) were produced at the lead-component interface with substantally lower strains at the board-lead solder joint.

Thermal load and dynamic load

Typical image obtained during reconstruction of a double-exposure hologram of a board subjected to localized thermal input is shown in Fig. 11. In this case, the surface mounted device was "attached" to the "back" side of the board in the upper right corner. Quantitative analysis of the fringe pattern shown in Fig. 11, as well as other fringe patterns shown in this section, were made by performing vertical and horizontal scans of the image. More specifically, the vertical scans were made along the component's left edge, along its centerline, and along its right edge. In a similar manner, horizontal scans were made along the horizontal centerline of the component, and along the upper edge of the component, unless otherwise specified.

Representative displacements of thermally loaded component, corresponding to the image

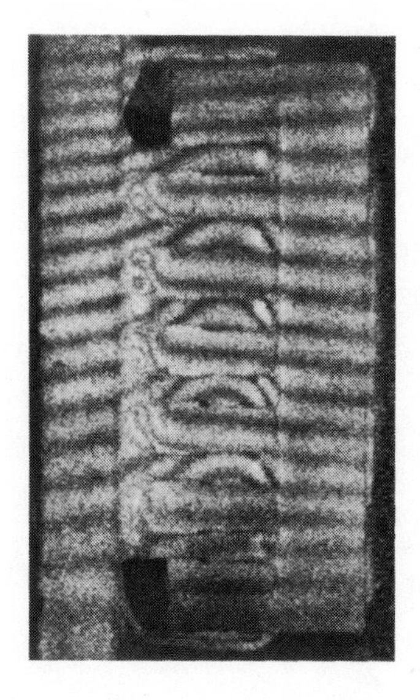

Fig. 9. A typical image produced during reconstruction of a double-exposure heterodyne hologram of a component experiencing flexural load.

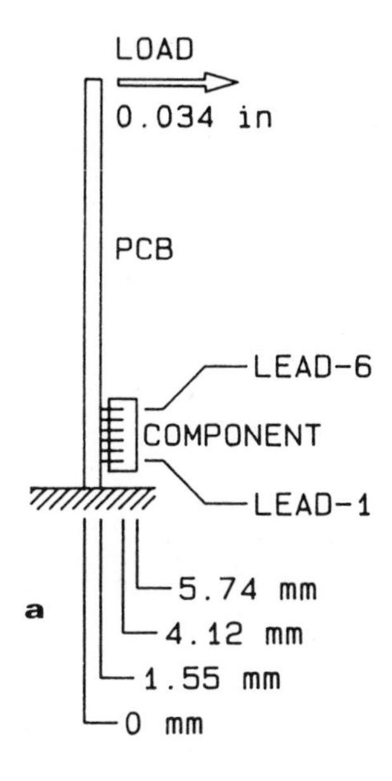

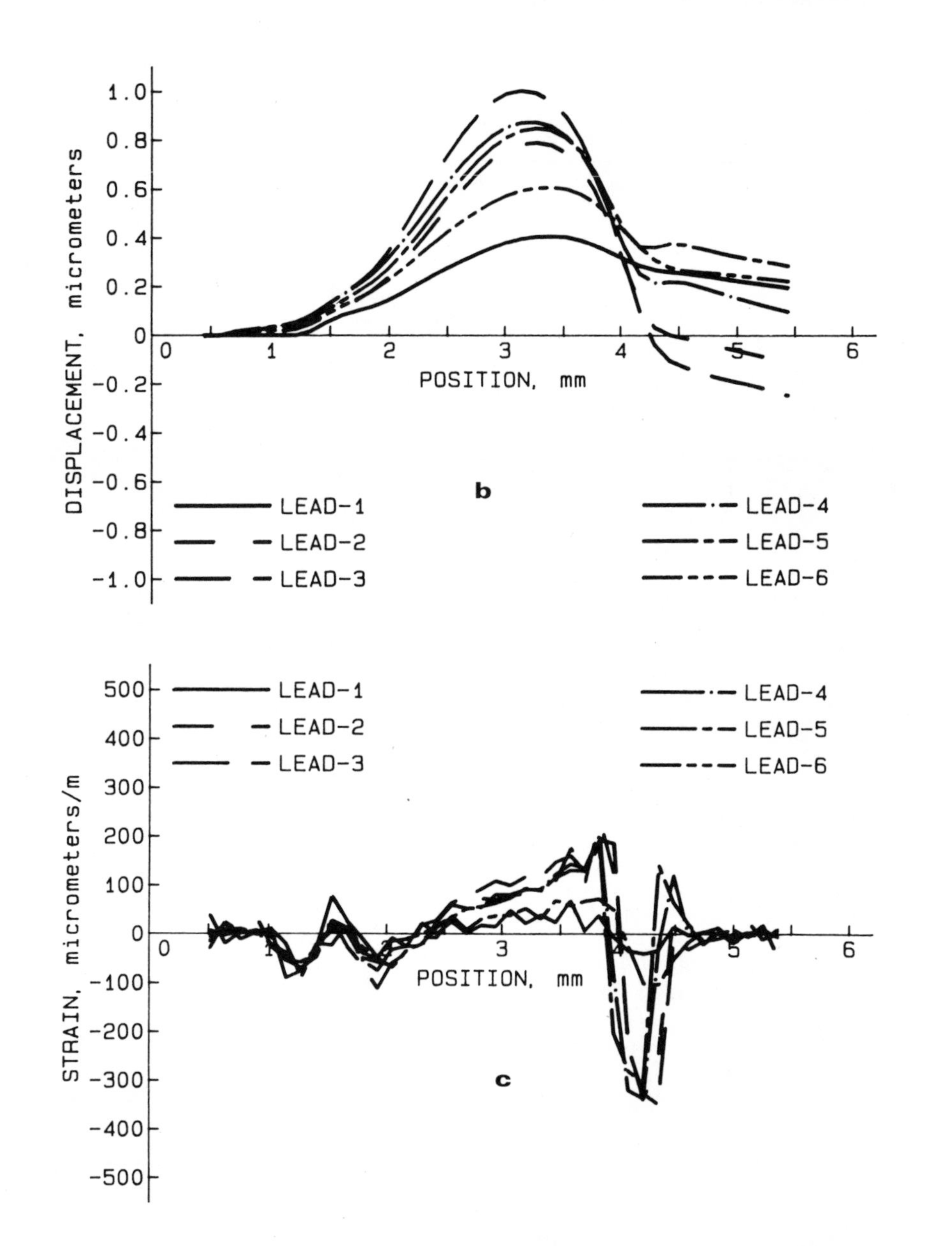

Fig. 10. Typical results obtained from a double-exposure heterodyne hologram of a loaded component: a) component geometry and loading condition, b) displacement versus position, c) strain versus position.

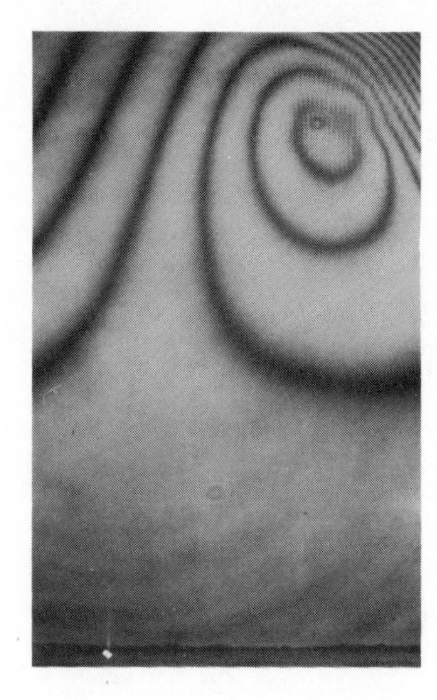

Fig. 11. A typical image obtained during reconstruction of a double-exposure hologram of a component subjected to a thermal load.

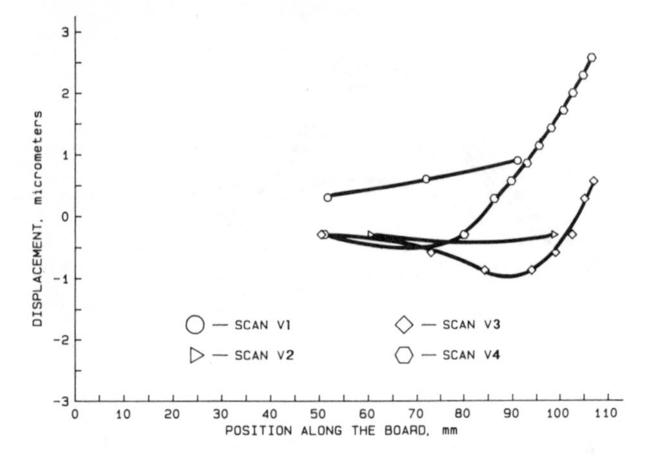

Fig. 12. Displacement versus position along the component determined from vertical scans of the image shown in Fig. 11: scan V1 is along the left edge of the board, scan V2 is along the central axis of the board, scan V3 is along the line through the center of the heated area, and scan V4 is along the right edge of the board.

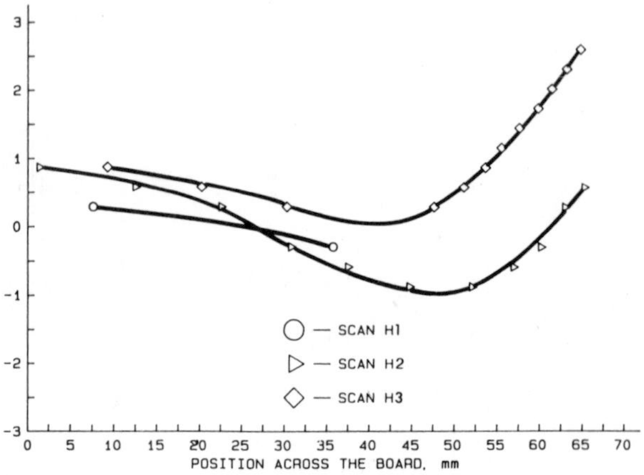

Fig. 13. Displacement versus position along the component, determined from horizontal scans of the image shown in Fig. 11: scan H1 is along the central axis of the board, scan H2 is along the axis through the heated area, and scan H3 is along the upper edge of the board.

of Fig. 11, are shown in Figs 12 and 13. These results indicate that displacements of a thermally loaded component ranged from -0.86 μm to 2.62 μm.

Figures 14 to 16 show time average holographic images of a component vibrating at its first bending more, first torsion mode, and second bending mode, respectively. The corresponding displacements versus position on the vibrating component are shown in Figs 17 to 20. The results shown in these figures indicate that mode shapes and amplitudes of displacement can be quantitatively determined from the time average holograms of vibrating components. More specifically, these results give displacements of the vibrating component from -1.17 μm to 3.07 μm, as a function of position on the component and the particular mode of vibration.

Conclusions

The results presented in this paper show that displacements and strains of small components can be measured using the methods of hologram interferometry.

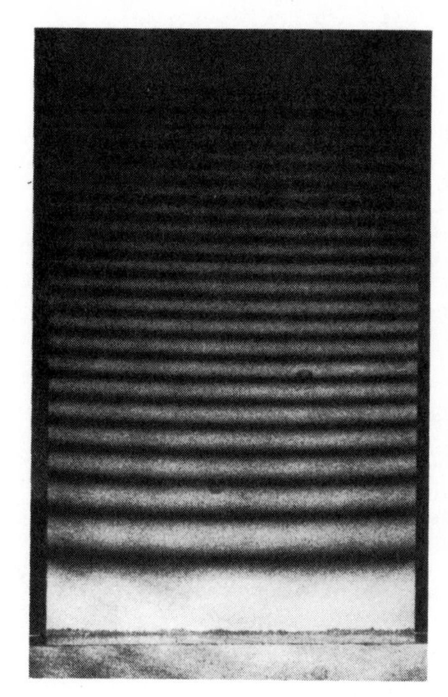

Fig. 14. Image obtained during reconstruction of a time average hologram of a component vibrating at its first bending mode.

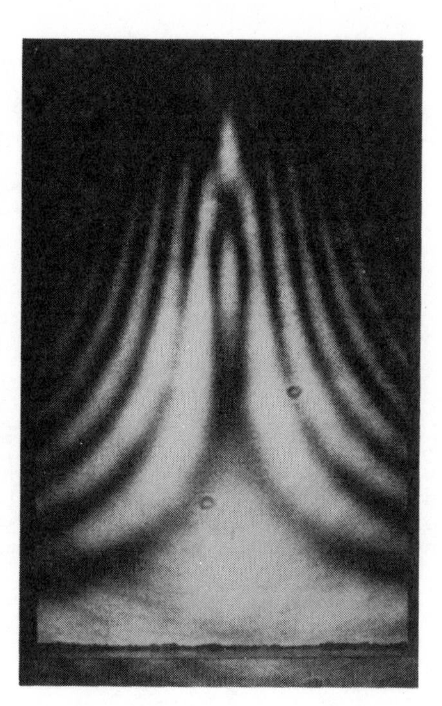

Fig. 15. Image obtained during reconstruction of a time average hologram of a component vibrating at its first torsion mode.

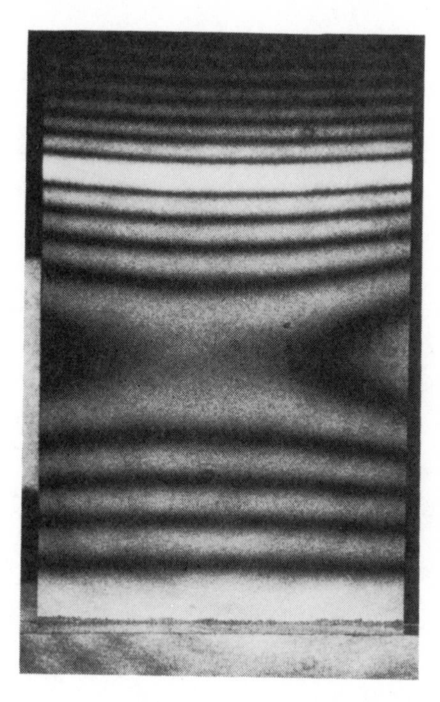

Fig. 16. Image obtained during reconstruction of a time average hologram of a component vibrating at its second bending mode.

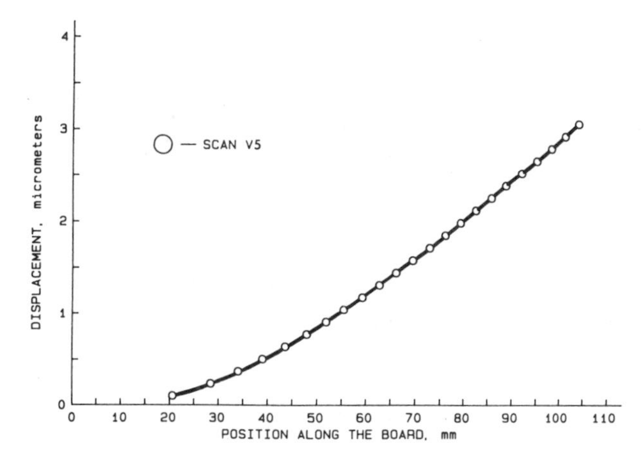

Fig. 17. Displacement versus position along the component, determined from the image shown in Fig. 14, vertical scan along the central axis of the board.

The methods of hologram interferometry allow accurate, non-invasive quantification of characteristics of small components. Procedures that allow mathematical interpretation of the fringe patterns, observed during reconstruction of holograms, are complex, but solvable with an aid of a digital computer.

Quantitative interpretation of the double-exposure heterodyne holograms shows that lead displacements on the order of 1.2 μm were obtained. Also, the data show that the component moves relative to the board as evidenced by the non-zero displacements at the lead-component interface. The corresponding strains were up to 540 μm/m.

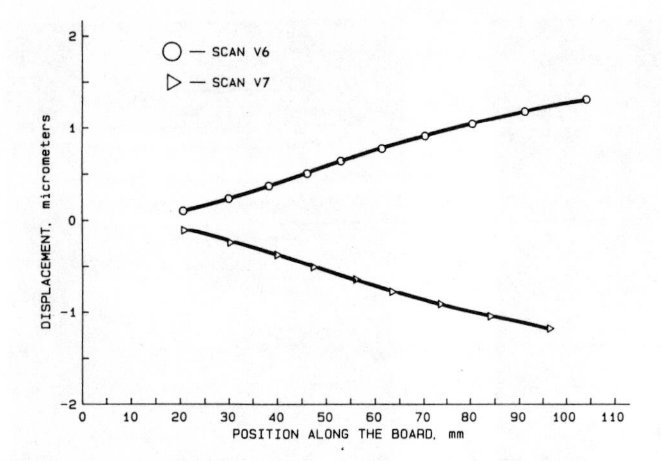

Fig. 18. Displacement versus position along the component, determined from vertical scans of the image shown in Fig. 15: scans V6 and V7 were made along the left edge and the right edge of the board, respectively.

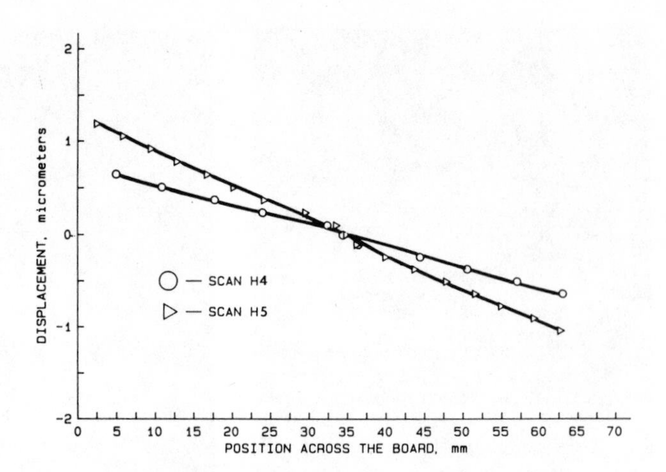

Fig. 19. Displacement versus position along the component, determined from horizontal scans of the image shown in Fig. 15: scans H4 and H5 were made along the central axis and along the upper edge of the board, respectively.

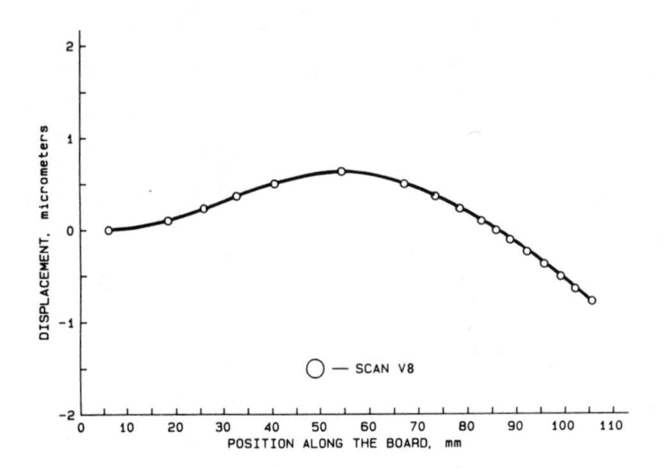

Fig. 20. Displacement versus position along the component, determined from the image shown in Fig. 16: scan along the vertical axis through the center of the board.

Also, current methods of hologram interferometry allow quantitative interpretation of holograms of vibrating components and components that are thermally loaded.

All in all, the results presented in this paper show that displacements and strains can be measured on small components. Furthermore, using the method of heterodyne hologram interferometry, these measurements can be made remotely in a non-invasive manner with high accuracy and precision, on the actual small components. These results on mechanical characteristics of the components, together with the results of studies on the components' response to thermal loads and dynamic excitation are, in turn, used as input parameters for an optimum design of small components.

References

1. Pryputniewicz, R. J., and Stetson, K. A., Fundamentals and Applications of Laser Speckle and Hologram Interferometry, Worcester Polytechnic Institute, Worcester, MA (1980).
2. Pryputniewicz, R. J., and Stetson, K. A., "Holographic Strain Analysis: Extension to Include Perspective," Appl. Opt., 15:725 (1976).

3. Stetson, K. A., "Effects of Beam Modulation on Fringe Loci and Localization in Time Average Hologram Interferometry," J. Opt. Soc. Am., 60:1378 (1970).
4. Pryputniewicz, R. J., "Time Average Holography in Vibration Analysis," Opt. Engrg., 24:1378 (1985).
5. Pryputniewicz, R. J., "Quantitative Interpretation of Time Average Holograms in Vibration Analysis," in print.
6. Pryputniewicz, R. J., "High Precision Hologrammetry," Int. Arch. Photogram., 24:377 (1982).
7. Pryputniewicz, R. J., "Holographic and Finite Element Studies of Vibrating Beams," SPIE-599 (1986).
8. Pryputniewicz, R. J., "Holographic Determination of Rigid-Body Motions," Appl. Opt., 18:1442 (1979).
9. Dändliker, R., Marom, E., and Mottier, F. M., "Two-Reference Beam Hologram Interferometry," J. Opt. Soc. Am., 66:23 (1976).
10. Schuman, W., and Dubas, M., Holographic Interferometry, Springer-Verlag, Berlin (1979).
11. Pryputniewicz, R. J., "Quantification of Holographic Interferograms: State of the Art Methods," Technical Digest, OSA, Washington, D. C. (1986).

* * *

Examples of holographic testing versus state-of-the-art in the medical device industry

James W. Wagner

Materials Science and Engineering Department
The Johns Hopkins University
34th and Charles Streets
Baltimore, Maryland
21218

Abstract

The medical device industry has seemed rather reluctant to integrate holographic technology into their product lines. While independent researchers have demonstrated the great potential for holography in imaging and display, it appears that holographic techniques may have the greater potential to solve some of the *in-vitro* testing and quality and process control problems peculiar to the medical device industry. Examples of these techniques include *in-vitro* testing of strain distributions surrounding bone plates, contouring for wear properties of artificial joints, and rapid nondestructive determination of leak rates in implantable electronics packages. With new advances in optics and electro-optics comes the hope that these and similar techniques may soon become integral parts of medical device manufacturing.

Introduction

The development of holographic techniques for medical applications can be grouped into one of four categories: clinical diagnostics, imaging and display, medical research, and industrial process/quality control. It is with regard to the last two categories that this paper will speak most directly. One should realize, however that research related to device development and techniques applied to process and quality control represents only a fraction of the activity surrounding the use of holography in medicine and biology. In the areas of imaging and diagnostics, for example, there have been advances in interference microscopy[1], pattern recognition[2], holographic ophthalmic cameras[3], and related diagnostic instrumentation. By far the most active area of development has been in the use of holography for stereo and pseudo-3D display of images acquired by x-ray and nuclear medicine techniques[4,5]. Likewise in medical research there has been wide spread use of holographic interferometry and contouring in the studies of the properties of bone and teeth[6].

As stated above, examples of holography in medical research aimed at medical device development or in medical device manufacturing process and quality control are somewhat less common. Never-the-less, holographic applications in these areas do exist and in some cases are challenging more conventional technologies. To illustrate this point, three examples will be discussed: *in-vitro* testing of metallic bone plates, wear measurements of orthopedic implant materials, and testing seal integrity of implant electronics. Finally, some comments on the outlook for holographic testing in the medical device industry will be presented.

Holographic Applications

The three examples to be discussed each represent an application of a different holographic technique. In order of their presentation they include holographic interferometry, contour and heterodyne holographic interferometry, and optical correlation. In each case, the continued use of the more conventional technology to provide these types of measurements remain more common in the industry than their holographic counterparts in spite of the apparent advantages of the holographic techniques. Some possible reasons for this will be discussed later.

Bone Plate Testing. In their simplest form, bone plates are metallic strips, perhaps 4 to 8 inches in length, drilled and counter-bored along their length in order to accept screws used to attach the plate to the bone. Generally made of stainless steel or a titanium alloy, they are used as short-term implants to approximate the ends of a fractured bone to help assure proper healing. In recent years, physicians and medical researchers have come to learn that, in performing their function of fixing the free ends of a fracture, bone plates also redistribute the stress through the fracture site. In many cases the bone callous which results from the healing process develops in a nearly stress-free environment. Consequently, this new bone tissue may be poorly organized and very weak. It is not uncommon for patients to refracture a bone within days after a bone plate is explanted. In order to help alleviate this problem, newer designs using more flexible structures and lower modulus materials are being investigated which provide fixation while still "sharing" some stress with the developing bone callous.

To investigate the stress distribution through the bone and bone plate combination, cadaver femers or tibiae are often sawn, plated, instrumented with strain gages, and subjected to bending and compressional loading. From the strain gage data, the performance of a particular bone plate design may be deduced. Studies of out-of-plane surface strain distributions are readily performed as well using holographic interferometry[7]. In the study cited, double exposure holograms were recorded before and after a load was applied to the test specimen. From the data obtained, differences in strain distributions for different bone plates were readily observed. Although this particular study is fairly old (reported in 1979), this type of work continues. In fact in 1985, one manufacturer released (and recalled) a new "modified stiffness" bone plate design for clinical studies.

Wear measurements of implant materials. Proper design and materials selection for the articulating surfaces of replacement joint prostheses requires an understanding of wear properties. Conventional stylus profilometers are useful only for metallic specimens which are nominally flat. Even then there is a possibility of scoring the surface so that further wear testing on the same specimen cannot be performed. For total knee and hip implants, it is in general true that one of the articulating surfaces is an alloy or ceramic while the other is a polymer or polymer matrix composite. In addition, these surfaces are machined with rather high curvatures- radii in the neighborhood of 0.5 to 1 inch. As a result, stylus measurements are not performed, in general.

Conventional wear testing of these components is never-the-less performed by the manufacturer by studying the wear particles which result from in-vitro testing. The device component to be tested is placed in a wear machine designed to simulate in-vivo service. The specimen itself is submerged in a bath of warm saline solution which simulates the implant environment. By circulating and filtering the solution, wear particles are recovered, examined, dried, and weighed. These techniques provide only an estimate of the wear volume without providing any indication of the distribution of the wear.

Two common holographic contouring techniques are the double wavelength and dual refractive index procedures[8]. Both can be used to make double exposure holographic interferograms which, upon reconstruction, generate an image of the specimen with superimposed contour fringes. Although both techniques have been employed for contouring implant devices, the dual refractive index procedure is used most often[9,10]. The double refractive index technique employs a conventional holographic set-up like the one shown in Figure 1. The object to be contoured is placed in a chamber with an optically flat glass window through which the object can be illuminated and viewed. The chamber is filled with a fluid of known refractive index and an initial exposure is made. After draining the chamber and refilling it with a fluid of a different index, a second exposure is recorded. The resulting reconstructed image has contour fringes whose spacings correspond to a surface height variation equal to one half the optical wavelength divided by the difference in refractive index between the two fluids. Often it is possible to get adequate fringe spacing simply by using air as the fluid within the chamber and changing the pressure between exposures. To the extent that one can control the refractive index of whatever fluid is used in the chamber, the contour interval may be varied continuously over a broad range from about 1.5 to 500microns. Figure 2 shows the contour of the tibial component of a knee prosthesis which was generated using the double refractive index method. In this case, two solutions of slightly different concentrations of ethanol in water were used.

Unfortunately, the holographic contouring techniques just described suffer from a dynamic range which is too small to permit direct application to the measurement of wear in the tibial component of the knee implant. Note in Figure 2 that while the fringes clearly show the general curvature of the knee "sockets", there is no indication of a gouge some 2mm wide, 0.5mm deep, and about 1cm long which was machines into the specimen before the contour hologram was recorded. While the contour fringe rate could be increased in an attempt to help detect the gouge, one is limited by the fact that the normal contours of the specimen may give rise to such large numbers of fringes that they can no longer be resolved or analyzed. Thus by increasing the fringe rate too much, one could actually lose sensitivity to surface defects in regions where the normal surface curvature is relatively high. Further, sub-fringe displacements may not be detected at all even on an otherwise flat surface. In other words, the ability to detect variations in surface contour is limited by the dynamic range of classical holographic interferometry. The lower sensitivity limit is set by the wavelength of the light and the refractive indices of the fluids used to generate the contours. The upper limit is determined by the highest fringe rate which can be resolved by the imaging system.

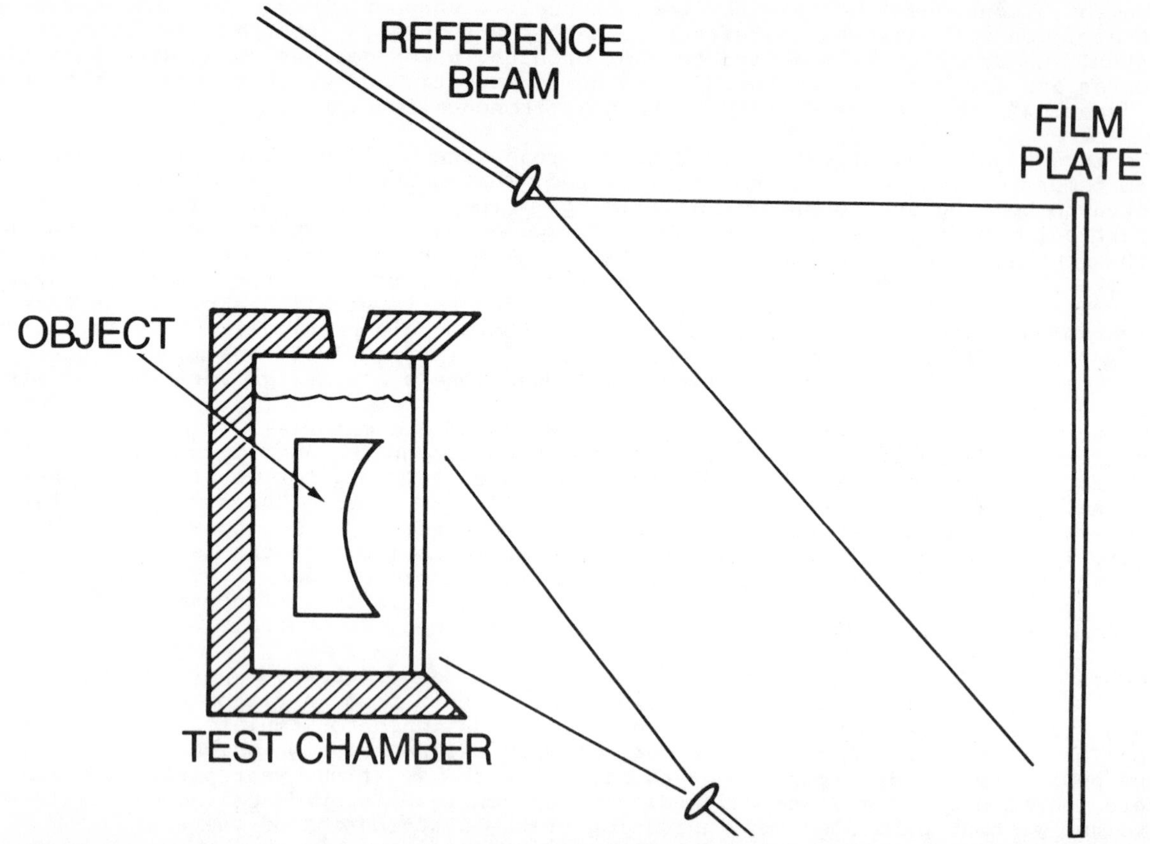

Figure 1: System for recording dual refractive index contour holograms.

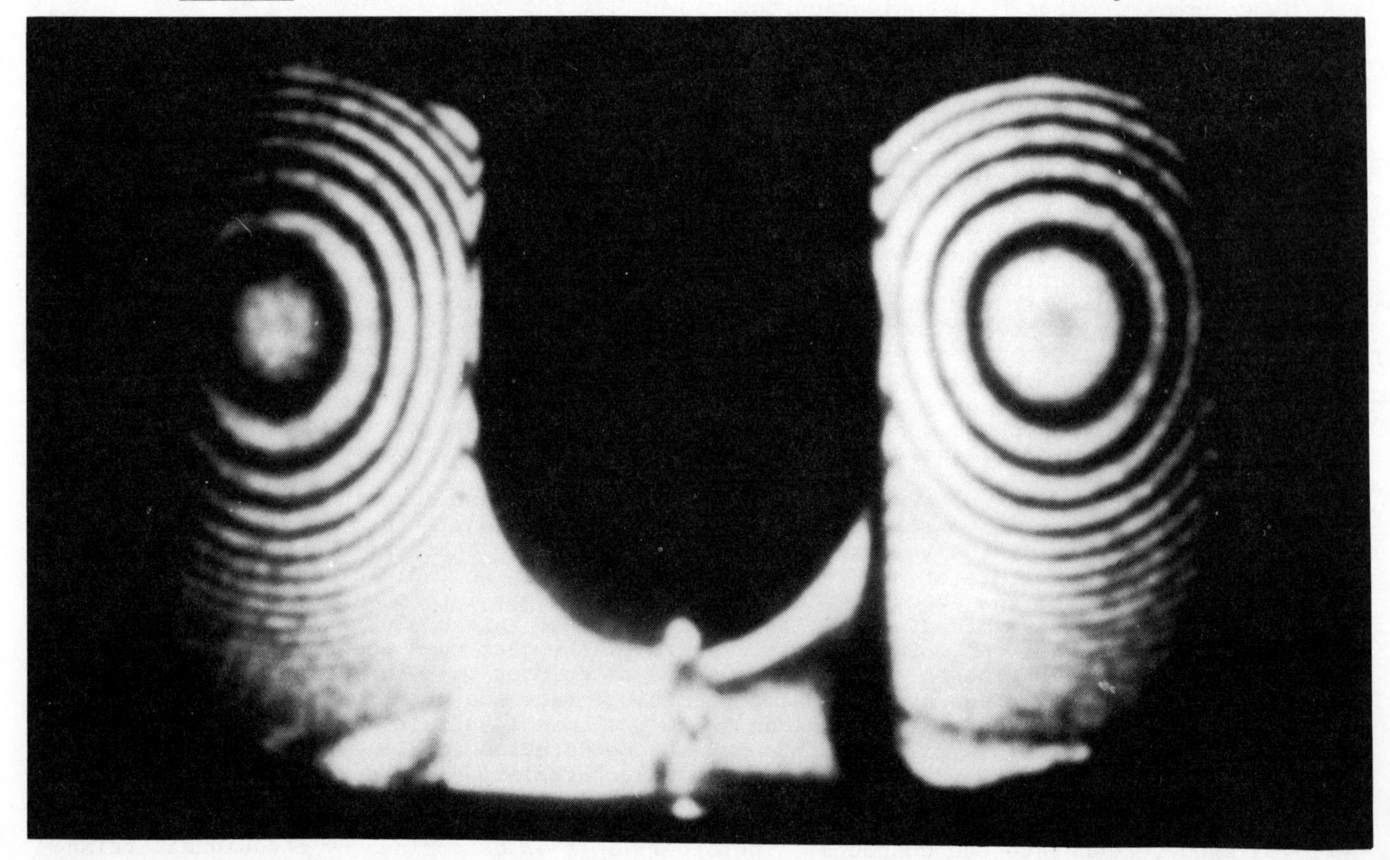

Figure 2: Contour hologram of the tibial component of a total knee prosthesis.

One method which has been used to overcome the limited dynamic range associated with contour holography of complex surfaces is a technique called heterodyne holographic interferometry[10]. To record a double exposure hologram for heterodyne analysis, a set-up such as the one diagrammed in Figure 3 is used. Note that a second reference beam has been added to the conventional recording geometry. Corresponding to each holographic exposure, first one, and then the other reference beam is used. Thus upon reconstruction, each reference beam reconstructs one image so that it is only when both beams illuminate the hologram that an interferogram is observed. If one of the two reconstructing beams is shifted to a frequency slightly different from that of the other, the previously observed stationary interference pattern will appear to precess over the reconstructed image of the object.

At shift frequencies on the order of 100kHz, the fringes appear to move so rapidly that they are no longer visible to the eye. If however, a lens is used to project the interferogram image onto a photodetector, the passing fringes will give rise to a sinusoidal output current at the 100kHz difference frequency. If a second detector is placed next to the first in the image plane, it too will produce a 100kHz sinusoidal output, but perhaps with some phase difference relative to the first signal. In fact, if the distance between the two photodetectors is exactly one-half of the fringe spacing observed in the stationary fringe pattern, then the phase difference between the two signals will be 180 degrees. Thus by using an electronic phasemeter to measure the phase difference between the two photodetector signals, one can determine the number of fringes between any two points on the image to some fraction of a fringe. Under proper conditions, phase determinations of better than 0.4 degrees can be made in this manner, thus permitting interpolation between fringes to 1/1000 of a fringe. Digital "quasi-heterodyne" techniques have also been used for analysis of double exposure, dual reference holograms. While easier to perform than conventional heterodyne analysis, the resolution of this technique is limited to about 1/100 of a fringe[11].

Figure 4 shows the results obtained when heterodyne analysis was applied to gouged surface of the knee prosthesis. In this case, one detector remained fixed while the other was scanned over the imaged surface. The resulting phase difference between the two signals was then plotted as a function of the scanned detector's position. Note that the gouge, which was not at all apparent in the static contour hologram shown in Figure 2 is readily discernible in Figure 4.

<u>Seal integrity of implantable electronics</u>. Implantable electronic devices include cardiac pacemakers, defibrillators, nerve stimulators, and programmable drug delivery systems. Most often they are constructed by mounting packages containing hybrid or monolithic microcircuits to a circuit board which is, in turn, housed in a sealed external package. While the internal packages are usually made from ceramic or kovar, the external package is most often constructed of titanium or one of its alloys (6% aluminum, 4% vanadium) and sealed using an electron beam or inert gas arc welding. Feedthroughs are ceramic or glass with molded epoxy strain relief structures bonded to the outside of the case. Hermeticity of these packages is desired in order to prevent the intrusion of moisture into the electronics. In the presence of moisture, and especially with surface contaminants, corrosive electrochemical reactions can take place literally destroying the electronic conductors and components within the device.

Standard testing procedures established by the military under and spelled out in military standard 883 are designed to help measure leak rates of sealed packages. While there are many types of leaks and leak mechanisms, packages can be separated into two categories- gross and fine leakers. A gross leaker is a package whose leak rate is greater than about 1E-4 atm-cc/sec. Fine leakers are generally those with leak rates smaller than 1E-7 atm-cc/sec. The middle range is somewhat ill-defined. Military standard tests in the gross leak range include bubble tests which are fairly qualitative in nature. The package to be tested is immersed in a pressurized container of a fluorocarbon solvent. Assuming that the package is a gross leaker, some of the solvent will leak into the package during this phase of the test. After a sufficient bomb time, the package is removed to a second bath containing a higher boiling point solvent and at an elevated temperature. At this point, the solvent within the package will boil causing solvent vapor to bubble through the package leaks to the surface of the test bath. Judging from the size of the bubble stream, an experienced technician can estimate the order of magnitude of the package leak.

Two primary techniques exist for making fine leak measurements. Both employ a tracer gas of some sort rather than a liquid solvent and in addition they tend to be more quantitative than the gross leak measurements. Again the first step is to bomb the packages under test in a pressure chamber filled either with helium or radioactive krypton. After the bomb period, each package is placed into a detection cell. For helium leak detection the cell is vented to a mass spectrometer to detect the concentration of helium within the cell. From the helium concentration the package leak rate is computed.

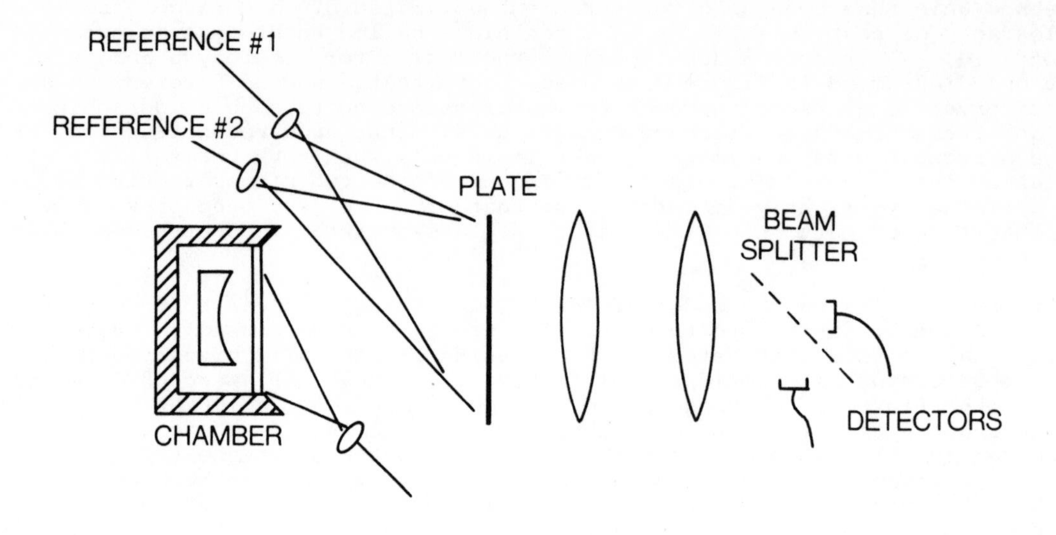

Figure 3: Recording and playback geometry for heterodyne holographic contouring.

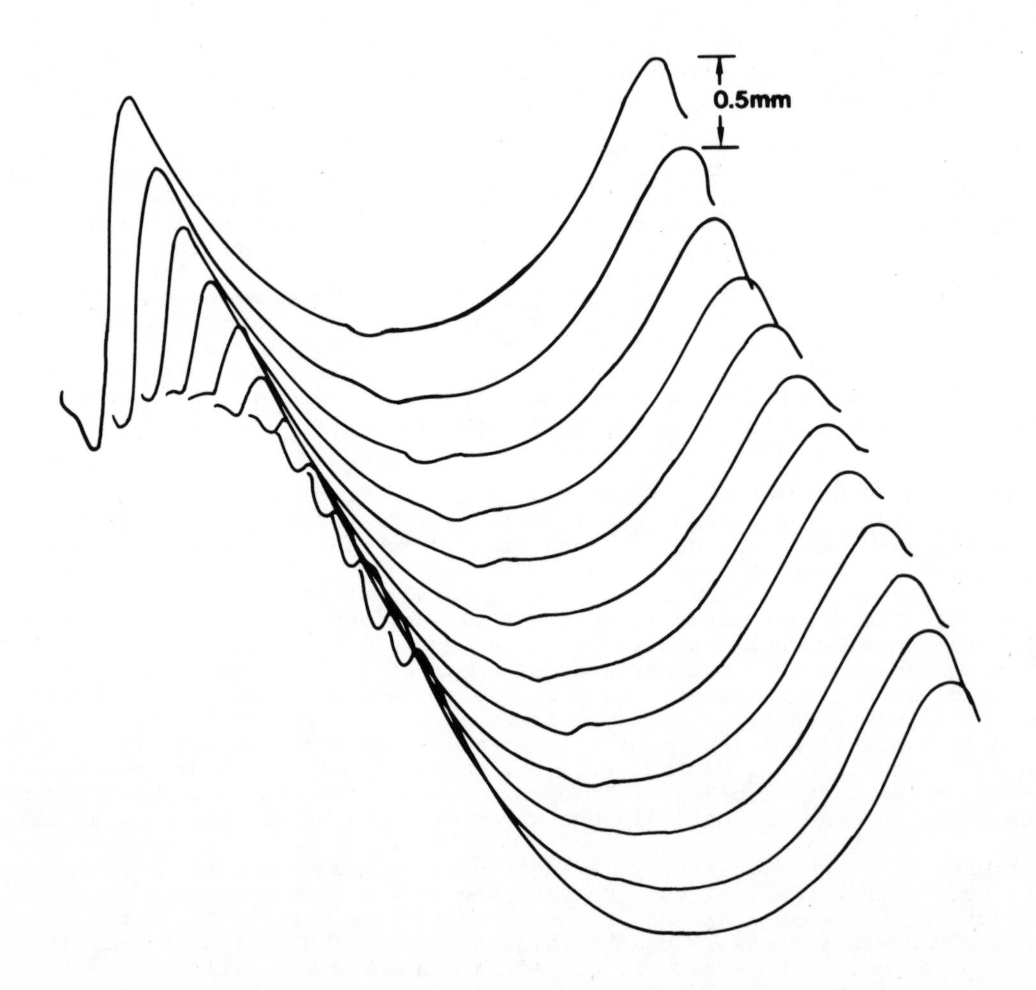

Figure 4: Surface profile of knee implant generated using heterodyne techniques.

Likewise, in the radioactive krypton system, the leak rate is computed from the scintillation counts from radiation emitted from the package. Large errors are often encountered as the leak rates approach those of gross leakers. Indeed it is possible to miss extremely gross leakers as most or all of the tracer gas may escape during the transfer from the bomb cell to the detection system. Errors may also be caused by the presence of polymers which absorb the tracer materials.

The holographic alternative to "mil standard" testing involves the use of optical correlation[12]. To understand how optical correlation may be used for leak testing, it is useful to remember that a correlation processor is nothing more than a pattern recognition system that is matched to a particular object shape and size. To measure the leak rate of a package, it is placed in a sealed test chamber fitted with a window to provide optical access to the package. A matched filter is then recorded using the holographic system shown in Figure 5. While the filter is being recorded, the pressure within the chamber is maintained at the same level as the atmospheric pressure under which the package has been stored. After development, the filter is replaced in the processor and the reference beam is blocked. Because the package matches the filter characteristics, a bright pinpoint of light will fall on the photomultiplier tube (PMT). If the package is replaced by another object or becomes deformed, however, the output intensity of the processor will fall and remain low until the original object is replaced or until the package shape is restored.

It is the ability of the correlation processor to "recognize" an object's shape that makes it useful as a means of detecting and measuring leak rates in packages. By this technique, one may detect the displacement and subsequent relaxation of the package surface resulting from an applied external pressure change. Figure 6 illustrates this displacement/relaxation phenomenon, showing a package placed in a sealed chamber wherein the pressure can be controlled. Initially, the air within both the chamber and the package are at atmospheric pressure (Figure 6a). To begin the test, the chamber pressure is increased by some amount, P, above atmospheric pressure. The package lid is immediately displaced at this time, and air begins to flow into the package through the leak (Figure 6b). As time passes, the pressure within the package equilibrates with that in the chamber, allowing the package lid to return to its original position (Figure 6c). A data acquisition system or chart recorder is used to record the output of the PMT throughout the test. When the pressure in the chamber is increased, the correlation signal drops to a minimum value. As the pressure within the package equilibrates with that inside the chamber, the correlation signal returns to its autocorrelation value. By measuring the time required for the signal to return and given the internal free volume of the package, one can compute the leak rate value.

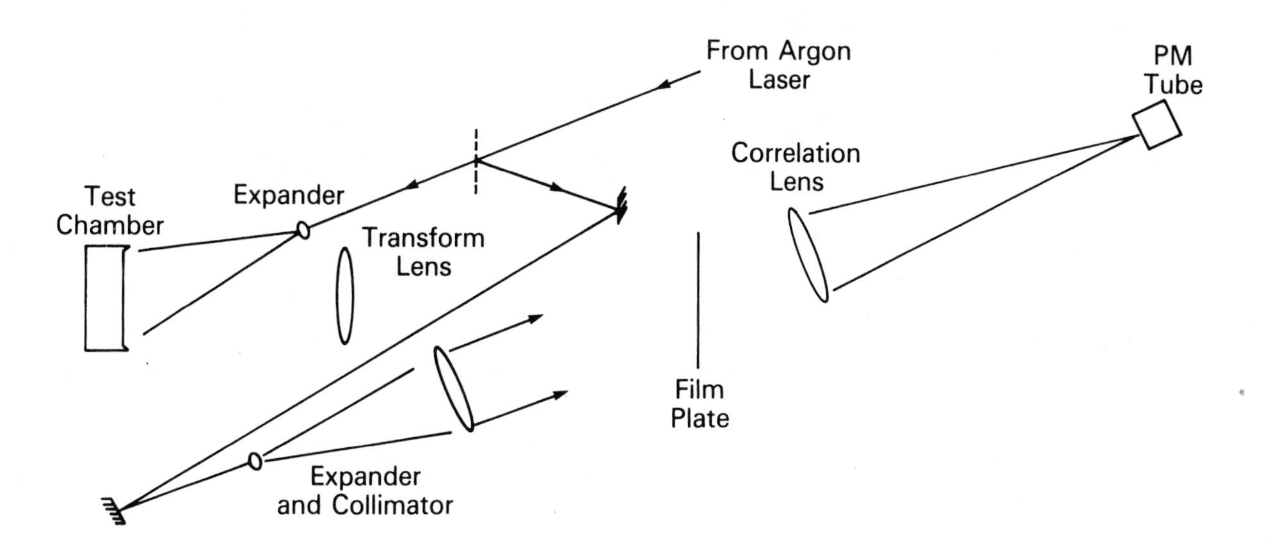

Figure 5: Optical correlation processor for leak rate measurements.

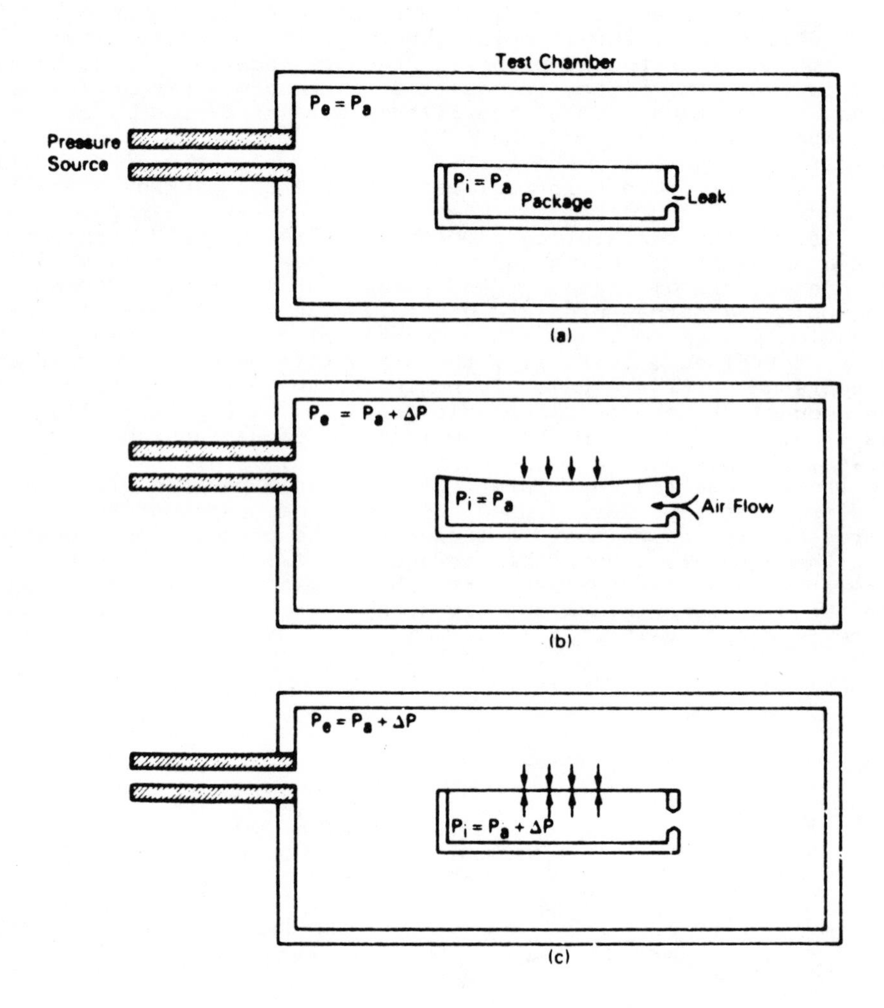

Figure 6: Response of a leaky package to a change in external pressure.

Optical correlation has been shown to provide an accurate means of detecting and measuring leak rates in sealed packages in the range from 1E-1 to 1E-6 atm-cc/sec in laboratory testing. Note that this range spans the gross leak and extends very near to the fine leak regime. With some modification in the testing procedure, it should be possible to extend these measurements well into the fine leak range. The technique offers several other advantages over more conventional tracer gas techniques that use helium or radioactive krypton gas. First, the optical technique suffers no loss in accuracy when polymer materials that may absorb tracer gasses are present either outside or within the package. Second, quantitative gross leak measurements with a zero miss rate are characteristics unique to this holographic approach. Finally, the optical correlation leak testing procedure can readily categorize certain types of leaks. For example, it is possible to determine whether a particular leak rate is the result of a single hole or of a region of very fine porosities. Such information may then be used to help pinpoint the processing step responsible for the leak.

Outlook for Holographic Testing

With one notable exception being the medical imaging community, it is has been true that in general medical device manufacturing practices have followed those developed first by the electronics and aerospace industries. Unfortunately, the transfer of technology from the high technology industries has not always been rapid or complete. Indeed with regard to manufacturing technology, the medical device industry represents a paradox of sorts. In the same manufacturing community, one finds, for example, the use of sophisticated machining and assembly processes associated with exotic alloys and, on the other hand, finds labor-intensive assembly line manufacturing often lacking adequate process or quality control. It is this later situation which one finds disconcerting in an industry whose priorities should include high reliability.

At a hearing before the Food and Drug Administration in 1977, one manufacturer of implantable cardiac pacemakers argued successfully that the state-of-the-art for sealing and inspecting seal integrity of electronics packages was, at that time, some four or five orders of magnitude poorer in medical device manufacture than in nonmedical electronics production! This opinion, supported by experts from the military and aerospace industries, came to light as a result of the manufacturer's voluntary recall of several thousand pacers suspected of being inadequately sealed to prevent the ingress of moisture into the sensitive electronics. When last surveyed in 1984, it was found that 100% inspection for seal integrity of pacemakers was still not as yet practiced by all manufacturers.

The fact that quality and process control procedures in much of the medical device manufacturing community have lagged behind those of their nonmedical, high-reliability counterparts can be understood, if not justified, by recalling some of the history and circumstances under which the modern industry has evolved. In the late 1960's and throughout the 70's, many small, single-product companies entered the medical device market. Low production volumes and frequent design changes prohibited investment into costly automated assembly facilities. Low volume demand typical of many medical products not only kept production costs high but also accounted for the high cost and, in some cases, limited availability of raw materials and OEM assemblies. (In the late 1970's one battery manufacturer who supplied "high reliability" batteries to producers of implantable electronics threatened to cease production of this particular product if medical manufacturers could not provide assurances that they would be protected from medical liability questions arising from the use of devices which employed their batteries.) As was mentioned earlier, these companies borrowed what technology they could from nonmedical manufacturers but seldom could afford to invest in the research and development of new quality or process control technologies to address problems peculiar to their products and processes. Even today after many of these small companies have merged or been bought up by other, larger companies, profits from medical device manufacture are affected by many of the same issues and, in some cases, further compromised by federal regulation and price restrictions imposed by insurance companies and third party providers.

From this understanding of the state of process and quality control testing in the medical device industry, two points emerge. First it is clear that there are real opportunities for new testing and sensor technologies for application in process control and 100% quality control inspection. The second point is that the development and implementation of new technologies for these purposes must take place under some fairly harsh economic restrictions. Thus, it is perhaps even more the case for the medical device industry than for other industries that only those technologies which show promise for immediate application can be considered for development. Once implemented, these techniques must not adversely affect production cost (by reduced throughput rate, for example). In addition, they must be able to accommodate product design changes with a minimum redevelopment cost.

Holographic methods must certainly be considered as candidates for application in medical device manufacturing. Indeed several holographic nondestructive testing techniques have been applied to medical device research and failure analysis and would appear to have direct application to quality control testing. Unfortunately, these techniques, although successful in their laboratory applications, have not as yet found their way to the manufacturing floor. With new advances in optics and electro-optics comes the hope that these and similar techniques may soon become integral parts of medical device manufacturing.

---

1 Snow, K., A holographic interference microscope in: Proc. of photographic science and engineering in medicine - equipment and techniques, July 1972, pp.39-49, Soc. Photographic Sci. Engrs., Washington,D.C.

2 Partin, J., et al., Autocorrelation of diatoms as a function of depth of focus, in: Holography in medicine and biology, ed. G. Von Bally, pp.73-76, Springer, Berlin, 1979.

3 Ohzu,H., Kawara, T., Applications of holography in ophthalmology, in: Holography in medicine and biology, ed. G. Von Bally, pp.133-146, Springer, Berlin, 1979.

4 Malacara, D., Optical and electronic processing of medical images, Prog. Opt., (22) pp.3-78, 1985.

5 Von Bally, G.(ed), Holography in medicine and biology, pp.83-130, Springer, Berlin, 1979.

6 ibid., pp.7-44 and 183-222.

7 Hanser, U., Quantitative evaluation of holographic deformation investigations in experimental orthopedics, in:Holography in medicine and biology, ed. G. Von Bally, pp.27-33, Springer, Berlin, 1979.

8 Varner, J., Holographic and moire surface contouring, in: Holographic nondestructive testing, ed. R. Erf, pp.105-147, Academic Press, New York, 1974.

9 Lalor M., Groves, D., and Atkinson, J., Holographic studies of wear in implant materials and devices, in: Holography in medicine and biology, ed. G. Von Bally, pp.20-26, Springer,Berlin, 1979.

10 Wagner JW, Gardner DJ, Heterodyne holographic contouring for wear measurement of orthopedic implants, Proceedings of the International Congress on Applications of Lasers and Electro-Optics, Los Angeles, CA (November 1983), Laser Institute of America, Toledo, OH (1984).

11 Hariharan, P., Quasi-heterodyne hologram interferometry, Opt. Engr., 24(4), pp.632-638, 1985.

12 Wagner, J. et al., Using optical correlation to measure leak rates in sealed packages, Appl. Opt.,21(20), pp.3702-3705, 1982.

CRITICAL REVIEW OF RECENT DEVELOPMENTS IN ELECTRONIC SPECKLE PATTERN INTERFEROMETRY

J R Tyrer

Department of Mechanical Engineering, Loughborough University of Technology
Loughborough, Leicestershire LE11 3TU, England

ABSTRACT

Electronic Speckle Pattern Interferometry (ESPI) is now fifteen years old. What has held it back in its development? Some recent developments enabling ESPI to become a commercial instrument capable of solving specific industrial tasks will be discussed. The use of this instrument to assist both the opto-mechanical engineer and the experimental engineer to help solve problems raised at product design level as well as later when "fire fighting" pre-production and in- situ crisis that require very short investigative response times.

1.0 INTRODUCTION

The use of holography gave the scientist and engineer the opportunity of using interferometric analysis on real everyday components over and above simple optical surfaces confined within specialist laboratories. The use of holographic interferometry (HI) has several advantages over conventional techniques:

(i) it is absolute in using the wavelength of the laser as its measuring base rather than a comparative technique such as photoelasticity or brittle lacquers.

(ii) it produces a whole field very high resolution analysis rather than specific point contacts.

A further major advantage is:

(iii) it is unobtrusive and does not require any surface applicants which can distort the information from the component under investigation.

HI therefore had the potential to give comparatively quick solutions to component problems and scientific investigations with relative ease. The ability to undertake a three dimensional investigation with the high displacement sensitivity provided by the laser attracted many to the field. The interferometric sensitivity proved to be a handicap which necessitated the building of special purpose laboratories with suitable rig design to enable valid test results to be produced. Many endured these problems and established test facilities capable of examining their workpieces to produce interferograms displaying suitable fringe patterns. The interpretation of these fringe patterns proved to be a further difficult and arduous task. Meanwhile the relative costs of suitable digital processing equipment led to this task being considered for semi automatic high speed analysis. Therefore specialist manufacturers were able to incorporate such facilities within production, though more likely, within development areas. Today the number of routine holographic end users is very small. Apart from these technological handicaps, the industrial inertia needed to accept new technology and the education of the general community to appreciate the advantages of such has as usual been very slow.

With the maturing of the technology, holography has found specific engineering niches and with it the developments of reliable emulsions, reusable thermoplastic cameras, longer life, low maintenance light sources to name but a few. Still the problem of fringe analysis exists though several groups claim degrees of success with the automation in this area. To produce a full displacement analysis requires at least three views of an object if space and laser power permit. Economies in these areas can introduce error functions which can, in certain circumstances, be as large as the measurements being made.

During the late 1960s work in Europe, and in particular at the National Physics Laboratory in England, had been investigating the phenomena of laser speckle. Considered by most holographers as the bane of coherent illumination, this "annoyance" can still relay information about a surface. The combination of the imaged speckle pattern and a reference wavefront to produce a phase referenced speckle pattern can be used in a similar way to holography. The speckle interferometer was used to visualise vibration patterns with the coarse interferograms blurring areas of movement to display the nodal lines to the observer. The use of double exposure photography to record two different positions of the object would display interference fringes identical in construction to a corresponding holographic study. The idea of linking this speckle interferometer with a television camera was the advantage that set apart this type of instrument from holography. The ability to capture images using a video system combined with enhancements achieved by subsequent electronic processing developed a new, more efficient instrument, called the Electronic Speckle Pattern Interferometer (ESPI). Rather than supply a series of references to many different journals, I would draw the readers' attention to a book covering this, "Holographic and Speckle Interferometry" (1983) by Jones and Wykes, as suitable for further reading and a source for references.

The subsequent development of ESPI in both the practical and theoretical areas has been investigated primarily by two major groups, one at Loughborough University of Technology under the leadership of the late Professor John Butters, and the second at Trondheim University under Ole Lokberg. This does not exclude the contributions made by other groups in Europe, US and Japan.

In this review paper I will consider the basic principles of ESPI, the different configurations, the applications and the industrial relevance now as commercial instruments become available.

2.0 BASIC PRINCIPLES OF ESPI

With reference to Figure 1.1, the basic optical configuration can be considered as a focussed image holographic system. The reference wavefront is mixed with the imaged wavefront using a beam splitter prior to the imaging sensor of the television camera. The object is illuminated usually with an expanding beam whose axis is close to that of the axis of the imaging lens. These conditions sensitise the system for displacement along the axis of the imaging lens, ie out of plane (a similar holographic arrangement results in the observer seeing the object within the reference beam). The size of the speckles is governed by the size of the imaging aperture, thus enabling the matching of the speckle with the resolution of the television camera imaging sensor. The intensity of the resulting speckle interferogram then contains three main terms:

$$I = I_1 + I_2 + \sqrt{2 I_1 I_2} \cos \phi$$

where I_1 and I_2 represent the object and reference intensity and ϕ the relative phase.

The interference term $2 \sqrt{I_1 I_2} \cos \phi$ is the signal carrier in the video system and therefore the DC terms of I_1 and I_2 can be filtered electronically. Rectification of the interference term will also enhance it. The enhanced signal can now be digitised to a minimum of 8 bit to avoid degradation before being stored in a digital frame store. Originally this was achieved using analogue video tape and was demonstrated by Butters and Leendertz[2].

If the object generating the speckle pattern moves away or toward the television camera the brightness of the interference term will vary cyclically from bright to dark to bright with every phase increment of π radians, or by $\lambda/2$ along this axis. Every speckle in the interferogram will undergo this cyclic variation independently since the phase of the light from each speckle varies randomly from speckle to speckle.

Every subsequent picture from the television camera undergoes similar processing, but bypasses the digital frame store and goes through an image inverter. Thus the addition of this new signal with the stored image results in image subtraction. The result is viewed on a television monitor after undergoing suitable reconfiguration into an analogue signal. One immediate advantage of such correlation subtraction is the removal of optical noise and intensity variations contained within the system. Problems of gross body movement resulting in the decorrelation of the speckle have been covered by Jones and Wykes[3]. The maximum number of fringes that can be easily identified across an object surface is approximately 40 and, whilst the system is capable of more, the fringe contrast begins to make visual perception difficult. Consequently the maximum displacement, using a Helium Neon laser, that can be considered at any one time is approximately 12μ. Displacements greater than this can be considered by simply readdressing the framestore at this maxima before continuing the loading of the component. This staircase loading can continue providing that a record of the stages is kept, allowing the overall displaced shape to eventually be produced. Being a correlation subtraction process Denby and Leendertz[4] realised the potential for reconfiguring the optics to provide a method of examining pure in-plane displacement. Effectively by illuminating the surface with parallel planes of light (produced from the interference of two opposing sources) decorrelation of the speckles would only occur if displacement took place across these planes of illumination, see Figure 2.1. A more useful experimental system is described in Figure 2.2.

To conclude this section it is therefore possible with one instrument to sensitise the optical arrangement to examine sequentially the three orthogonal displacement vectors. The ability to analyse displacement in just one vector in isolation is possible and can be considered as an advantage over holography.

3.0 DISPLACEMENT ANALYSIS

This can be broken down into two main sub-sections: 3.1 Static Analysis which examines two distinct object conditions and 3.2 Dynamic Analysis which maps the surface movement between two positions during the object motion.

3.1 Static Analysis

The basic sensitivity of the system is shown in Figures 3.1 and 3.2, where (d) describes the displacement needed to produce a dark fringe in a subtracted speckle pattern. For a more complete description of the system sensitivity see Wykes[4]. The fringes represent contours of constant displacement in the sub-micron region from 0.25 μm to 0.5 μm, dependent upon the laser wavelength and optical arrangement used.

To consider static applications of ESPI, four different types of loading are considered, they are: pressure, thermal (convective heat transfer), point mechanical and microscopic.

3.1.1 Pressure Loading

The result in Figure 3.3 is of a prototype commercial honeycomb panel subject to two different pressure states (the difference is of the order of 2-3 psi). The internal pressure difference within the individual cells of the honeycomb highlights areas of adhesive debonding, highlighting these as the smaller diameter contour patterns. Similar testing has been undertaken on pneumatic tyres along the lines of the holographic tyre testing, but using ESPI the possibility of providing automatic analysis of these contour patterns now exists.

3.1.2 Thermal Loading

Figure 3.4 presents an interesting study of the distribution within a domestic incandescent light bulb. The ability to map the changes in refractive index within a medium combined with the greatly reduced exposure time for the television equipment enable studies of transients and thermal instabilities far more easily than with holography.

3.1.3 Mechanical Point Load

In order to satisfy national standards components must be examined in specified ways, figure 3.5 demonstrates a plastic floor moulding (0.9 m x 0.9 m) being subjected to a point load. This loading arrangement represents a human operator sitting on a chair, such that the total load is being put through one chair leg. The component is used as flooring within computer rooms and enables the cable runs to be laid underneath without interfering with passageways etc. The study was run in parallel with a finite element analysis and both were used to produce a complete theoretical and experimental investigation of the component.

3.1.4 Microscopic Studies

Work by Herbert[6] examined the crack tip displacements due to plastic zone formation in both composites and plastics. The area of investigation was typically approximately $1mm^2$, and the component could be loaded from an initial state right through to ultimate fracture. Here surface magnifications of up to x100 were used to investigate linear elastic fracture mechanics. One major advantage of ESPI in this type of analysis is the ability for immediate and continued updating of the initial surface reference state such that the experiment can be built up from rest to ultimate fracture.

3.2 Dynamic Analysis

The other major branch of experimental analysis for ESPI is in the area of vibration studies. This can be further broken down into two major sub-categories:

(i) Laboratory analysis - continuous wave lasers
(ii) On-site analysis - pulsed lasers

3.2.1 Laboratory Based Dynamic Analysis

The stability requirement to record a hologram is that all components including the surrounding environment must remain stable to at least $\lambda/8$. The recording time is a function of the recording medium sensitivity, component size and available laser power. With a continuous wave laser the required exposure time is usually in the order of seconds or tens of seconds for holograms and consequently the required stability during that exposure must be better than 0.1 μm to ensure a high quality image. With a television camera in ESPI, the inherent gain in sensitivity of the imaging tube enables the exposure to take 1/25 sec (1/30 sec for NTSC standards in USA), the aperture of imaging lens can be used to optimise the light level.

To undertake vibration analysis the component is excited at one of its natural resonant frequencies. The vibrating component is isolated from the optical system to ensure the measures taken to establish an experimental set-up, capable of maintaining the $\lambda/8$ requirements, are not now defeated by sympathetic rig oscillations. Acoustic coupling between the component and optics must also be guarded against. These measures are usual for large structures oscillated at low frequency (DC - 1 kHz), above this, the response will be damped by the basic optical table etc.

The component is left oscillating during the recording time and the fringe function is no longer $\cos^2$ but the characteristic J_o^2 (zero order Bessel function), the harmonic case has been considered in depth by Stetson and Powell. From this reference, the resulting image can be considered as

$$I(x',y') \propto J_o^2 \,[4\pi/\lambda \; a_o \; (x,y)]$$

where $I(x',y')$ is the imaged intensity of the sinusoidally vibrating object and a_o is the amplitude of vibration at position (x,y). The electronic processing described earlier assists with the visualisation of the higher order fringes, the high pass filtering removes the DC term from the reference beam and the rectification enables approximately 10 higher order fringes to be observed. In this time-averaged mode of operation the dynamic range of ESPI does not approach that of holography, it is restricted by the noise performance, gamma correction and the speckle size. This limitation has led to the development of noise reduction techniques covered later in this paper.

With time averaged recording the phase information is lost. The fringe patterns display amplitude fringe maps that are easy to interpret because areas of no movement show up as bright fringes. These nodal lines are displayed at the full intensity of the television system. The brightness of the displacement fringes will be described by the J_o^2 function envelope but will have maxima where a_o is 0.25, 0.45, 0.66 etc, the fringes represent contours of constant vibration amplitude, approximately equal to an integer number of $\lambda/4$.

3.2.1.1 Phase Modulation

To overcome the problems of poor fringe visibility and loss of phase information, phase modulation within the reference beam can be introduced. This was reported by Lokberg and Hogmoen[8]. The simplest way of achieving this is to replace one of the passive reflective elements within the interferometer with one capable of being vibrated under both amplitude and frequency control. The object vibrates with amplitude $a_o(x,y)$ at point x,y and has an associated phase of $0_o(x,y)$. The vibrating mirror is oscillated with the same frequency f as the object but with an amplitude a_r and phase 0_r.

With reference to figure 1.1, if the angle between the object illumination and observation is > 5-10° then the image will be

$$I(x',y') \;\; \alpha J_o^2[4\pi/\pi[a_o^2(x,y) + a_r^2 - 2a_o(x,y)\; a_r \cos(0_o(x,y) - 0_r)]^{1/2}]$$

Therefore the maximum value will be reached when the phase and amplitude of the vibrating mirror match those of the object point (x,y). The value of this when trying to analyse complex fringe patterns is that areas of movement that are in phase will be easily identified. Consequently the phase relationship of these sites with adjacent areas of vibration can be determined by the phase change introduced within the reference beam. This technique is not only of value in vibration analysis but also in determining dynamic modulii of materials as reported by Rowland[9]. The use of phase modulation can be seen in figure 3.7 where the relative phase between the two adjacent antinodes is 180°.

The usual method of exciting this mirror is to adhere it onto a piezoelectric crystal which is bonded onto the mirror support. Therefore this vibrating mirror is now a dynamic structure with its own associated resonant characteristics. Therefore the electronics controlling the amplitude and phase of vibrating mirror must take into account the system response. Tilt errors can also be introduced if care is not taken with the choice of the mirror within the interferometer. To remove the tilt and dynamic problems of the mirror an electro-optic transmission element is used, the penalties are higher driving voltages and cost.

For in-plane analysis one of the mirrors in figure 2.1 can be vibrated.

3.2.1.2 Stroboscopic Analysis

The previous two sections have averaged the component response over the operating time of the television camera. If the component response is sampled at specific points then a different function can be used to describe the object motion. With large displacements (2 μm and above) the Bessel function has reduced the fringe contrast to such an extent that observation is made too difficult. The introduction of stroboscopic illumination originally reported by Pederson, Lokberg and Forre[10] changed the fringe function to a simple $\cos^2$ function. Therefore the fringe visibility is uniform over the whole object area.

In order to generate the stroboscopic action a continuous wave laser is chopped to produce a series of light pulses. The simplest methods of achieving this are: with mechanical rotating disc, electro-optic or acousto-optic choppers. The use of external cavity devices such as cavity dumpers have been tried but cost, alignment and stability requirements are prohibitive for anything other than fundamental and very specialist requirements, for general engineering purposes these external devices are unsuitable.

As with stroboscopic holographic interferometry, the light pulses are usually synchronised with the peaks of displacement. Therefore the light modulation is at twice the frequency of the object vibration. The pulse duration is at least 1/10th of the object vibration period. If the object motion produces too many fringes for good fringe contrast it is possible to work on sections of the sinusoidal response curve other than the peaks. Usually this is confined to the "linear region" of the sinusoid as shown in figure 3.8.

The resulting image will be described by

$$I\,(x,y)\ \alpha \cos^2[(4\pi/\lambda)\ a_o(x,y)]$$

this assumes the same illumination conditions are used as in section 3.2.1.1.

With stroboscopic illumination and noise reduction techniques it has been possible to image speckle fringes over a surface of 5 pixels width. This suggests the system is capable of imaging over 100 fringes across the television screen (the digital frame stores and television equipment were working at 512 x 512 pixels) there is nothing to suggest the system could not work with fringes of 3 pixels width, further reductions would probably not be acceptable because of aliasing.

Unfortunately because of the light reduction suffered in chopping the laser (in view of the practical problems associated with external cavity dumpers) stroboscopic ESPI usually requires an argon ion laser. Frequency doubled YAG lasers have been successfully used at Loughborough to generate stroboscopic illumination though here the pulse duration was typically 10-20 nsec. This work is more completely covered in the next section.

3.2.2 On-Site Analysis using Double Pulsed Lasers

Pulsed laser ESPI was originally developed by Cookson, Butters and Pollard[11] working with ruby lasers. The performance of this equipment was limited by the pulsed lasers then available, subsequently this work was developed by the author to incorporate frequency doubled YAG lasers which offered further advantages over ruby based systems.

3.2.2.1 Pulsed Ruby Laser ESPI

The use of the imaging tube of the television camera to store and add two speckle interferograms was originally proposed by Pollard. The basic operating scheme for this type of ESPI is described in Figure 3.9. With double pulsed holography the recording medium, usually silver halide (maximum sensitivity of holographic materials), is very forgiving in terms of the relative intensity of the two laser pulses. That is to say a successful hologram can be produced even when the pulse intensities are not equal. With ESPI, however, the television camera is usually operating at the top of the imaging tube gain curve and any slight variation is likely to exceed the dynamic range of the imaging tube and produce no result. This places a constraint upon the quality of the ruby laser pulses. Due to the inherent inefficiency of the ruby lasing medium, heating occurs within the ruby rods during each operation. This heating effects the laser pulse and therefore stabilisation of the laser prior to each firing is required. Consequently instead of the laser repetition rate being greater than 10 per minute, it is practically reduced to 1 per minute. With the addition concept the camera field coils are switched off, the first laser pulse is synchronised to the object motion as described in Figure 3.10. Any laser pulse build up times (typically 1 ms) can be accommodated by the first variable delay such that the laser fires on the peak of displacement of the next oscillation. The pulse separation is determined by the period of the object oscillation but for maximum displacement this is /2 and is controlled by the second variable delay. Immediately after the second pulse the camera field coils are switched on and the combined interferogram read off the faceplate of the imaging tube. If the pulse separation is greater than 5 msec then the persistance of the standard vidicons and chalnicons will be exceeded and longer persistance tubes will be required. The image is then filtered, rectified, digitised and stored in the same manner as in figure 1.1. With this type of operation there is no need for the subtraction system to produce the necessary fringe information. It can however be used if the background optical noise is stored in a second frame store and the interferogram subtracted from this to enhance the quality of the fringes.

As with stroboscopic ESPI if the displacement is in excess of say 30-40 fringes then the "linear region" shown in Figure 3.8 can be used. For pulse separations of between 1 μs-1 ms, two pulses can be extracted from a single fluorescence of the ruby rod by double pulsing the Q-switch. The shortest interval between pulses is determined by the drive electronics to the pockels cell and the build up of sufficient energy within the ruby rod. The longest interval between pulses is determined by the length of the flashlamp pulse, this is typically 800 μs -1 ms. To balance the energy of the two pulses the delay between the flashlamp trigger and the Q-switch, the first Q-switch pulse voltage, the supplied energy to the flashlamps and the second Q-switch pulse voltage must all be controlled. These parameters select two optimum balanced pulses within the fluorescence envelope of one ruby pulse.

For pulse separations of 1 ms-5 it is necessary to fire the flashlamps twice. This is achieved by a second flashlamp capacitor bank which is charged simultaneously with the first, each bank is then used for one pulse. Caution must be exercised when working in the 1 ms-5 ms region when reduced energy is needed for the second pulse because the flashlamps will still be in a partially ionised condition. For most large structures the period of oscillation can be between DC-1 kHz with most work being between 5-200 Hz. Fortunately the Department of Mechanical Engineering has two such lasers, unfortunately the commercial pulsed ruby laser manufacturers deem these "specials" and subsequently impose large financial penalties.

For pulse separations greater than 5 sec, the recharging time within the capacitor charging system is sufficiently short enough to enable a second pulse to be produced.

3.2.2.2 Double Pulsed, Frequency Doubled YAG Laser ESPI

The industrial demand for on-site inspection using HI and ESPI as been restrained due to a suitable pulsed laser being made available. The pulsed ruby laser is a very large specialist device needing a large capital investment and skilled engineers to use and maintain it. Fortunately the development of YAG lasers specifically for industrial material processing has been such that turn-key, compact and ruggedised lasers are now commonplace. It was therefore a natural progression for the incorporation of such a laser into the speckle interferometer.

The YAG laser is inherently much more efficient and can therefore work with a greatly reduced power supply than the comparable ruby laser. Further the repetition rate of the laser can be much higher without the degradation of the light output due to reduced heating of the lasing medium. The obvious repetition rate to operate the laser is synchronous with the television system. For the UK, CCIR standards apply at 25 Hz, for the USA the NTSC standards are at 30 Hz. Both television systems operate on a 2:1 interface and to maximise fringe quality and reduce flicker, 50 and 60 Hz respectively should be used.

The laser made available could operate up to a maximum of 40 Hz (due to the design of the power supply drive electronics and not because of any optical limitations) though present work operates with lasers capable of repetition rates in excess of 60 Hz. The laser operated at a repetition rate of 25 Hz and was synchronised with the television system, thereby performing as a 'continuous' pulsed laser system. Using a harmonic doubling crystal the YAG laser output is 530 nm i.e. within the green part of the visible spectrum.

The design of the optical chassis of the laser enabled the primary wavelength (1.06 m) to be filtered and dumped so as not to present any potential safety hazard. These two features (the repetition rate and wavelength) of the YAG laser enabled the interferometer to be set up and operated with the ease of a conventional continuous wave laser based interferometer. The television camera used incorporated an extended red sensitive chalnicon imaging tube which enables it to work for both ruby (694 nm) and frequency doubled YAG (530 nm) pulsed lasers. The pulse to pulse quality of the YAG laser was such that the ESPI system could be operated as either an addition system, as described in section 3.2.2.1, or in a quasi-subtraction mode similar to the original description in section 2.0. The ability to store and subtract the optical noise generated within he interferometer yields considerable improvement to the fringe quality because spatial filtering cannot be used to clean up the object beam. This is because of the use of bi-concave beam expanding lenses to overcome the energy density propblems of air breakdown, material damage etc resulting from the focussing of conventional beam expansion. Therefore to subtract a reference condition from the double pulsed interferogram enhances the results which are displayed via a subsequent image store (either a second digital frame store or a video tape). A more complete description of this work was presented by Tyrer[12] at an earlier SPIE conference.

3.2.2.3 Fringe Analysis of Double Pulsed Interferograms

The first problem in the interpretation of double pulsed or stroboscopic fringe patterns is the determination of the zero order fringes. This is required to identify the nodal lines or areas of no displacement. With stroboscopic analysis the answer is to switch the stroboscopic operation off and work in the conventional time-averaged mode. However with a double pulsed system the fringes are of equal intensity and thus do not exhibit bright zero order fringes. The use of "quasi time-averaged" double pulsed HI reported by Gordon[13] is a simple technique to identify these zero order fringes. The Q-switch of the laser is operated such that the fixed Q of the ruby produces two longer duration pulses. This technique was applied to double pulsed ESPI and although it reduced fringe visibility the results showed an increased brightness along the nodal lines (on a vibrating speaker). Thus with the zero order defined the system reverted to conventional operation and thus identification could be made to the fringe field during interpretation. Relative phase delay between the laser system and the vibrating target is also needed, an example of this with pulsed holography was produced in an earlier paper[14].

4.0 RECENT IMPROVEMENTS

Ole Lokberg[15] put forward a paper with the controversial title 'ESPI - The Ultimate Holographic Tool for Vibration Analysis' and in the concluding remarks stated "The future acceptance of ESPI depends on how well it can compete with conventional holographic systems" and "It is unlikely, however, that holographic recording and display in the near future will obtain ESPI's combination of real-time capabilities, short exposure, high repetition rate".

End user comments have been similar, in that for ESPI to succeed as an engineering tool the fringe quality must be as good as with HI and a high degree of automated fringe analysis is required. This section will attempt to demonstrate that these requirements are being satisfied.

4.1 Vibration Fringe Enhancement

With conventional image processing noise reduction techniques, integration of the picture reduces random noise and enhances the actual image quality. Unfortunately with ESPI the speckle pattern, which would normally be considered as noise, is the signal carrier. With vibration analysis the fringe function and object detail is independent of the speckle pattern. The brightness and position of the individual speckles on the object surface is a function of the object illumination. Therefore if several interferograms are subjected to a variation in the object illumination and are integrated in an image store, the results displayed will show the stationary fringes enhanced and the background speckle pattern averaged out. Work at Loughborough initially reported by Davies, Montgomery and Tyrer[15] has been going on for some time optimising these conditions for storage within video and computer memories. Lokberg[17] has reported similar work using photography as the image store and Montgomery[18], using a video storage tube. Typical results are shown in Figure 4.1 here applied to a motor car engine vibration study for the optimised location of an engine predetonation (knock) sensor.

4.2 Use of Zoom Imaging Lenses

The basic optical arrangement for an out of plane sensitive ESPI is detailed on Figure 4.1. A major advantage of this layout is the ability to incorporate miniature format (35 mm) photographic lenses. With a fixed back focal length for single lens reflex cameras, the combination optics for the interferometer can be included in the space usually reserved for the camera mirror and shutter. Thus photographic zoom lenses can be incorporated to produce an ESPI which can examine a whole structure initially then zoom in to the specific areas of interest, identified by this initial study. A pan and tilt arrangement can be incorporated either by tripod mounting of the interferometer or use of a mirror on the object beam and imaging beam. Results of such a zoom lens are also shown in Figure 4.1.

4.3 Incorporation of Reference Beam Path Matching Compensation Leg

Work at Loughborough has refined the optical arrangement to minimise optical surfaces and maximise the object illumination, a performance indicator of this has been a study on a flat square surface of side length 1.1m, painted white and illuminated using a 15 mW helium neon laser. Object size and distance from the interferometer is constrained by the coherence length of the laser. Therefore when using a helium neon laser a multipass variable reference beam compensation leg has been designed and ruggedised. Depending upon the particular object requirements a 6, 8, 12 or 16 pass arrangement, with a typical maximum leg length of 300 mm can be used. Objects of several metres in diameter can be illuminated with a suitably powerful laser (usually Argon ion) externally mounted. This combined with imaging lenses, ranging in focal length from 30 mm - 250 mm, enable large or small engineering components to be examined with the minimum of object disturbance. This greatly reduces the required experimental time needed for a complete component analysis.

All these modifications to the original systems have been incorporated into a commercial system marketed by Ealing Electro Optics under the trade name of 'Vidispec'. A view of this equipment working on a large motor car engine and sub-frame can be seen in Figure 4.2. To illuminate the object a 5 watt argon ion laser was used, this laser is suspended underneath the optical table and a periscope arrangement used for input to the interferometer. Due to the object complexity and surface reflectance the on-board 10 mW helium neon laser was insufficient to examine the complete structure.

4.4 Contouring by ESPI

Initial work carried out using ESPI for contouring an object surface was carried out by Butters, Jones and Wykes[19,20] using a dual wavelength illumination approach. Recent work by Bergquist and Montgomery[21] using a rotating object beam and Winther and Slettemoen[22] using three point illumination enable a single wavelength to be used with variable contour interval. This work is beyond the scope of this paper, suffice to say it demonstrates a further application of ESPI and that a surface contour map is necessary for automatic computer fringe analysis.

5.0 COMPUTER BASED FRINGE ANALYSIS

Early work in this field was primarily aimed toward vibration analysis where ESPI has a considerable operating advantage over all other experimental techniques. The use of phase modulation enabled unambiguous fringe determination and early work in this area was undertaken by Koyuncu and Cookson[23] to semi-automate the data acquisition. The incorporation of this work into a commercially available image processing device was undertaken by Hurden[24]. This work was not fully automated requiring interactive fringe tracing with a light pen from the operator. Varman and Wykes[25] then improved the noise reduction algorithms and began the development of fringe tracking routines. This is now much easier with the improvements in fringe contrast discussed earlier. The work of Henry at Loughborough was used in a general applications paper by Montgomery and Tyrer[26]; he has been able to ruggedise the fringe tracking routines enabling a fringe field to be mapped into the computer in less than 30 seconds on a PDP 11-23, see Figure 4.3. Presently he is aiming to incorporate an array processor to further reduce this time to 1 sec.

The use of heterodyming and phase stepping are receiving the greatest effort at Loughborougn. Presently Kerr is using a 1024 x 1024 image processor with a front end digital pipe line processor to develop high speed software and synthesis front end hardware to further reduce the total processing time. This work is beyond the scope of this paper but will be the subject of a paper to be published shortly.

6.0 CONCLUDING REMARKS

Several attempts have been made to commercialise ESPI. The dramatic improvements in digital electronic equipment with associated cost reductions now enable the electronics associated with the equipment to be boxed in a small turnkey package. The development work by Roulstone and Bramley has produced ruggedised optical hardware which is capable of being transported to an industrial location and perform immediately. The involvement of large electro-optical equipment manufacturers with all necessary production and support skills now provide industry with a suitable interferometer capable of quantifiable experimental analysis on real objects in an industrial environment. Present development work with pulsed YAG lasers, diode lasers, fibre optics, contouring and automated fringe analysis will further improve and diversify the potential areas of industrial applications.

Holography has found limited industrial application and is used in certain engineering problem solving laboratories, ESPI (or TV holography) with its operating advantages over conventional holography will increase this situation. I shall end on a controversial note and raise the question, was Holographic Interferometry a stepping stone for Electronic Speckle Pattern Interferometry?

6.1 Acknowledgements

The author would like to acknowledge the guidance and motivation of the late Professor John Butters. Also the total cooperation and dedication of the 'Optics Group' at the Department of Mechanical Engineering; the active support of the SERC in funding this work presently as well as over the past 15 years and various industrial sponsors.

REFERENCES

1. Jones, R and Wykes, C. 'Holographic Speckle Interferometry', CUP 1983.
2. Butters, J N and Leendertz, J A. 1971 Jnl Measurement and Control 4, 349.
3. Jones, R and Wykes C. 1977, Optica Acta 24, No 5, 533-550.
4. Denby, D and Leendertz, J A. 1974. Jnl of Strain Analysis, 9, No 1, 17-25.
5. Wykes, C. 1982. Optical Engineering, 21, No 3, 400-406.

6. Herbert, D P. 1983, Optics and Lasers in Engineering, 4, 229-239.
7. Stetson, K A and Powell, R L. 1965, J Opt Soc Am, 55, 1593.
8. Lokberg, O J and Hogmoen, K. 1976, Jnl Phys E, Vol. 9, 847.
9. Rowland A C. 1985. Proc RPS and CEGB, 'Holographic Measurement, Speckle and Allied Phenomena, London.
10. Pederson, H M, Lokberg, O J and Forre, B M. 1974, Opt Com, 12, No 4, 425.
11. Cookson, T J, Butters, J N and Pollard, H C. 1978, Opt & Laser Tech, June, 119.
12. Tyrer, J R. 1985, Proc SPIE 599, Cannes (in print).
13. Gordon, A L, 1985., Optics & Lasers in Engineering, 6, 25-33.
14. Tyrer, J R. 1985, Proc SPIE 523, Los Angeles, 360-364.
15. Lokberg, O J, 1984, J Acoust Soc Am, 75, 6, 1783-1791.
16. Davies, J C, Montgomery, P C, Tyrer, J R. 1985, Proc ISATA, Graz, 73-92.
17. Lokberg, O J. 1984, ICO-13 Conference Digest, Japan.
18. Montgomery, P C. 1985, Proc SPIE 599, Cannes (in print).
19. Jones, R, Butters, J N. 1975, Jnl Phys E, Vol 8, 231-234.
20. Jones, R and Wykes, C. 1978, Optica Acta, Vol 25, 6, 449-472.
21. Bergquist, B D and Montgomery, P C. 1985, Proc SPIE 599, Cannes (in print).
22. Winther, S and Slettemoen, G A. 1984, Proc SPIE 473, Budapest, 44-47.
23. Koyuncu, B. and Cookson, T J. 1980, Jnl Phys E, 13, 106.
24. Hurden, A P M. 1982, Opt & Laser Tech. 2, 21.
25. Varman, P and Wykes, C. 1982, Opt & Lasers in Eng, 3, 87.
26. Montgomery, P C and Tyrer, J R, 1983, LIM2 Proc, Birmingham.

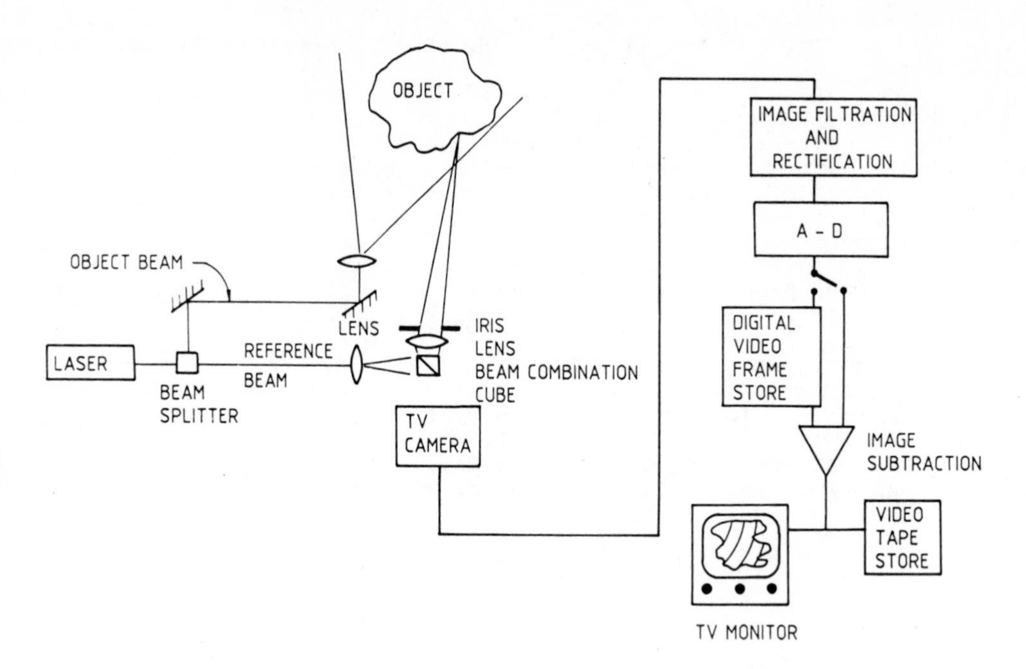

FIG. 1.1 SCHEMATIC FOR THE OPTICAL AND ELECTRICAL CONFIGURATION FOR AN OUT OF PLANE SENSITIVE ELECTRONIC SPECKLE PATTERN INTERFEROMETER (E.S.P.I.)

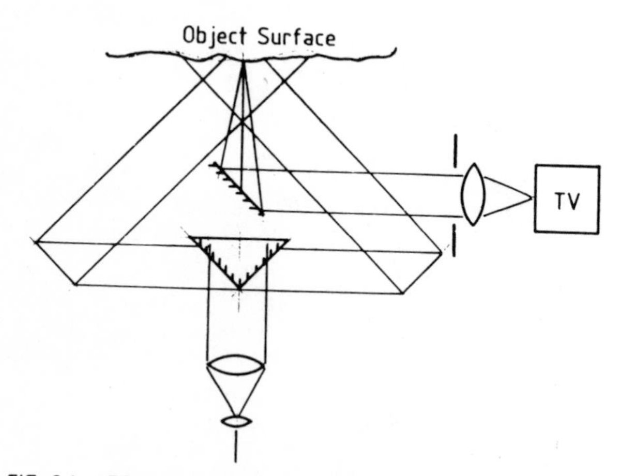

FIG. 2.1 ARRANGEMENT FOR IN-PLANE SENSITIVE SPECKLE PATTERN INTERFEROMETER

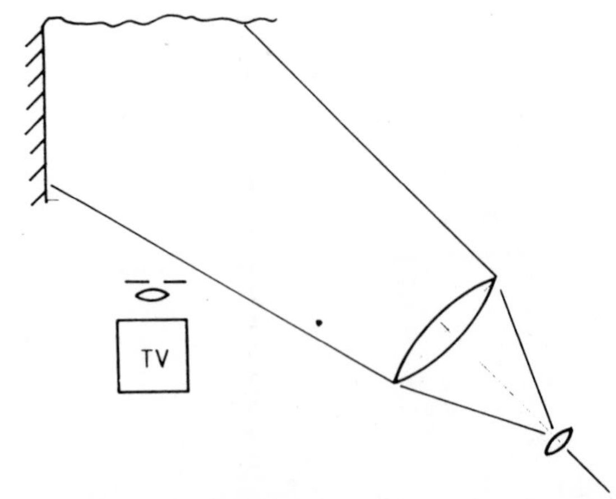

FIG.2.2 PRACTICLE ARRANGEMENT FOR IN-PLANE SYSTEM

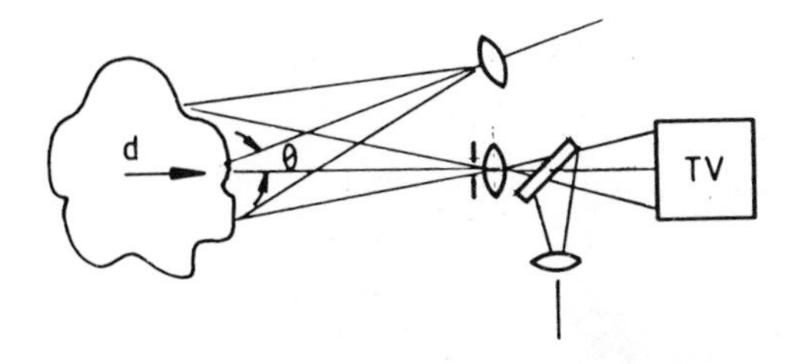

FIG, 3.1 SENSITIVITY OF OUT OF PLANE INTERFEROMETER

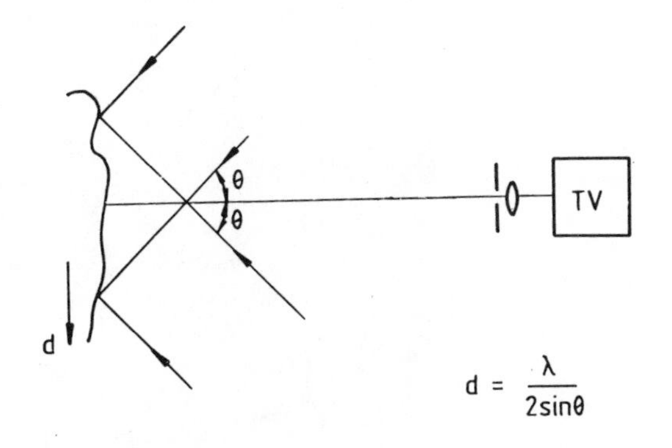

FIG, 3.2 SENSITIVITY OF IN-PLANE INTERFEROMETER

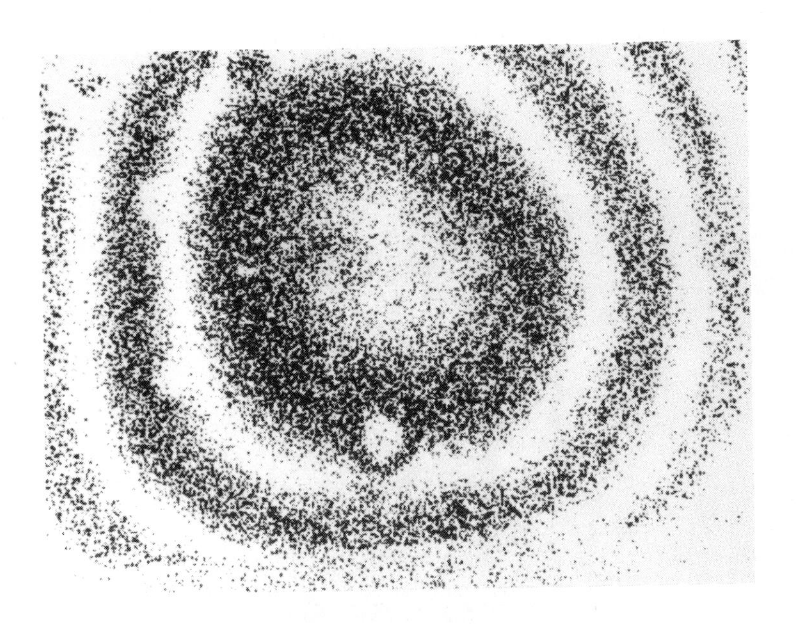

Fig. 3.3. Laminated honeycomb panel examined between two pressure states, the change in pressure highlights areas of adhesive debonding. (Courtesy of P. Montgomery).

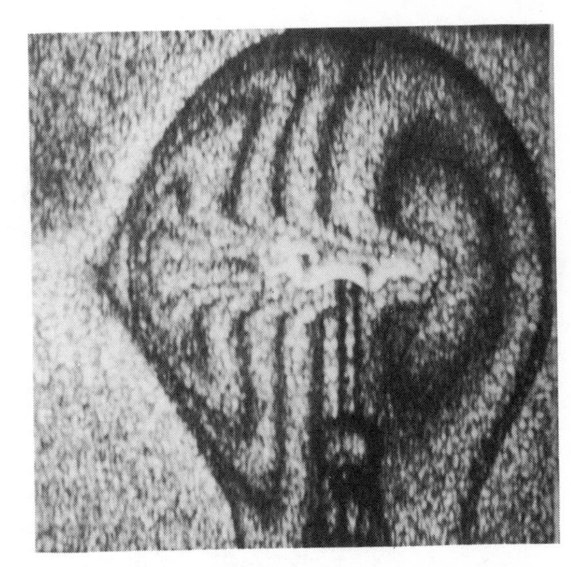

Fig. 3.4. The use of ESPI to visualise convective heat flow in a domestic light bulb.

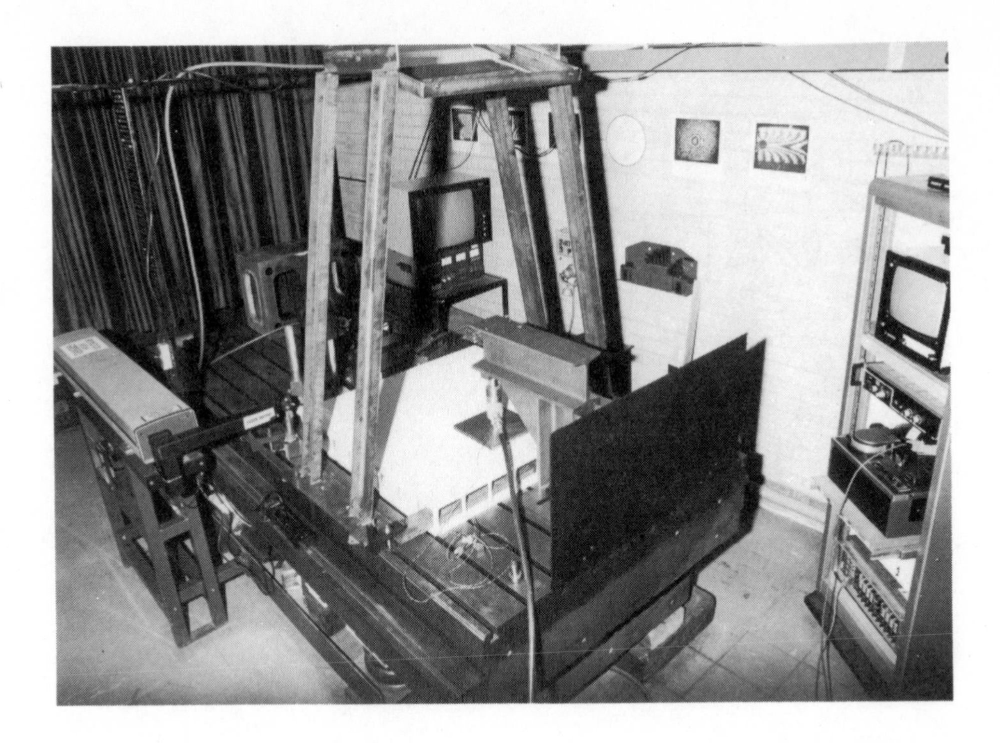

Fig. 3.5. The loading arrangement and typical results for a large area (0.9m x 0.9m) panel investigation.

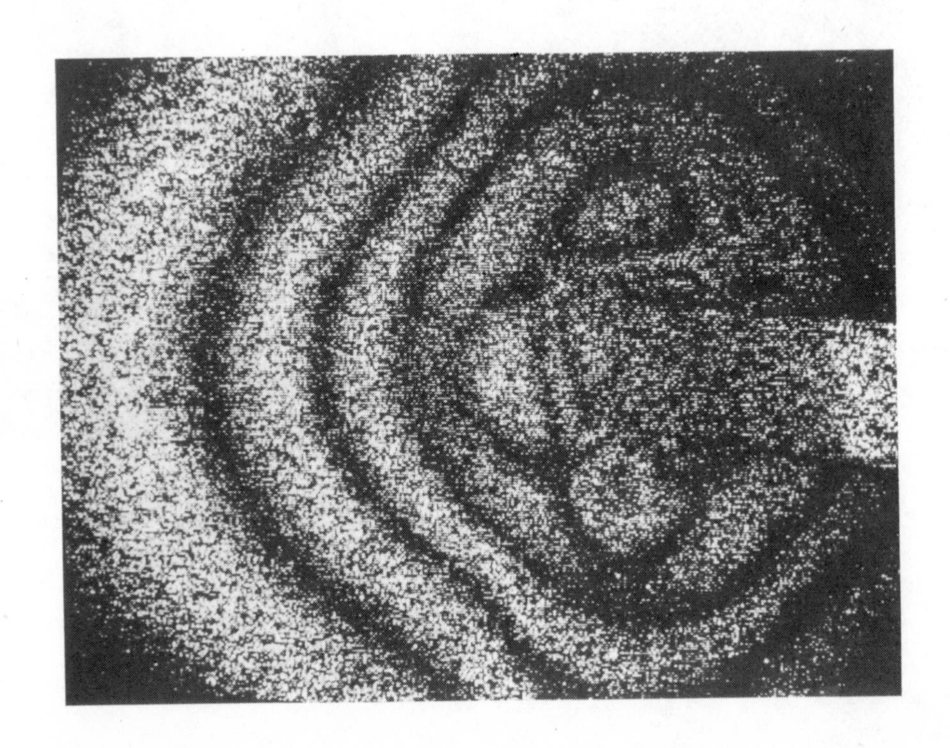

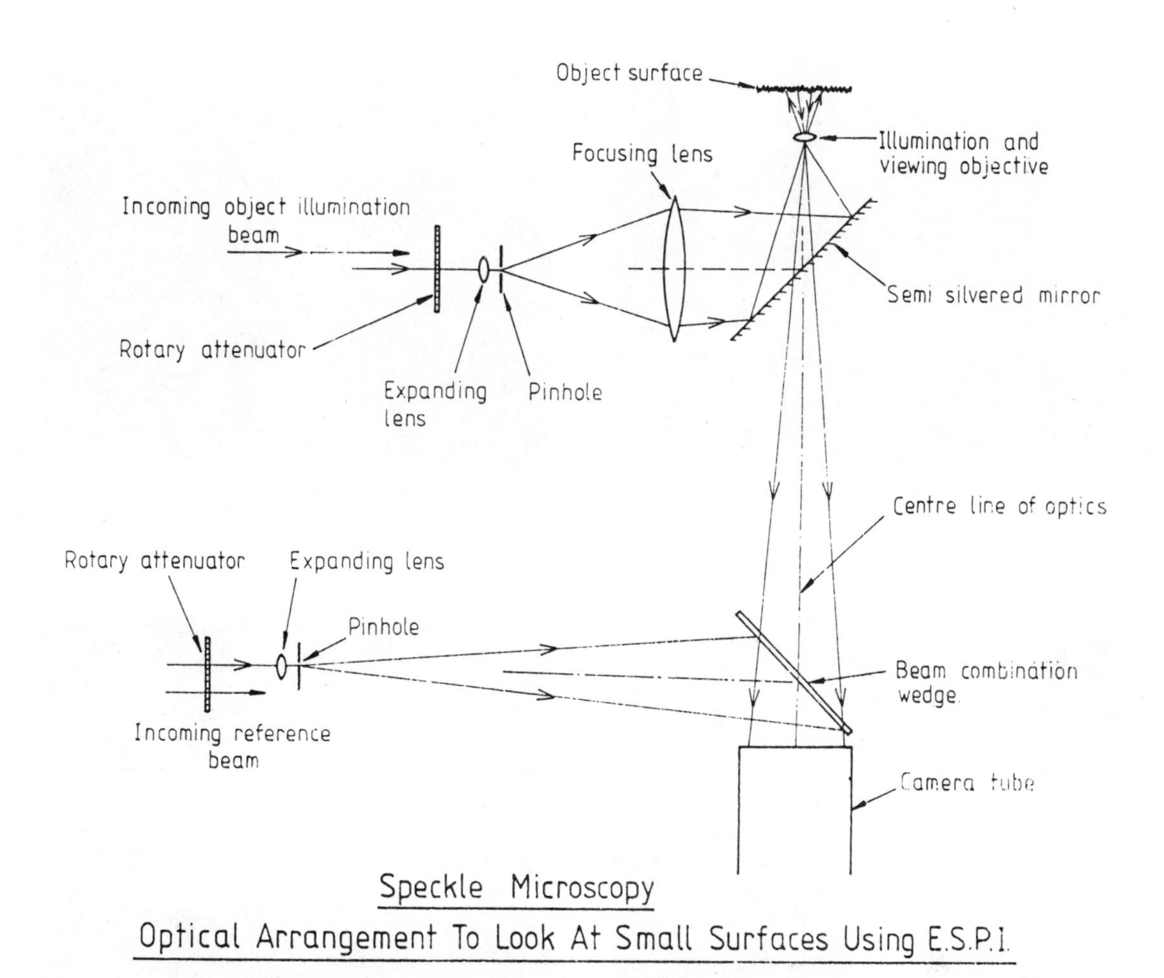

Fig. 3.6. Schematic and results for investigation over an area of $\sim 1mm^2$. (Courtesy of D.P. Herbert).

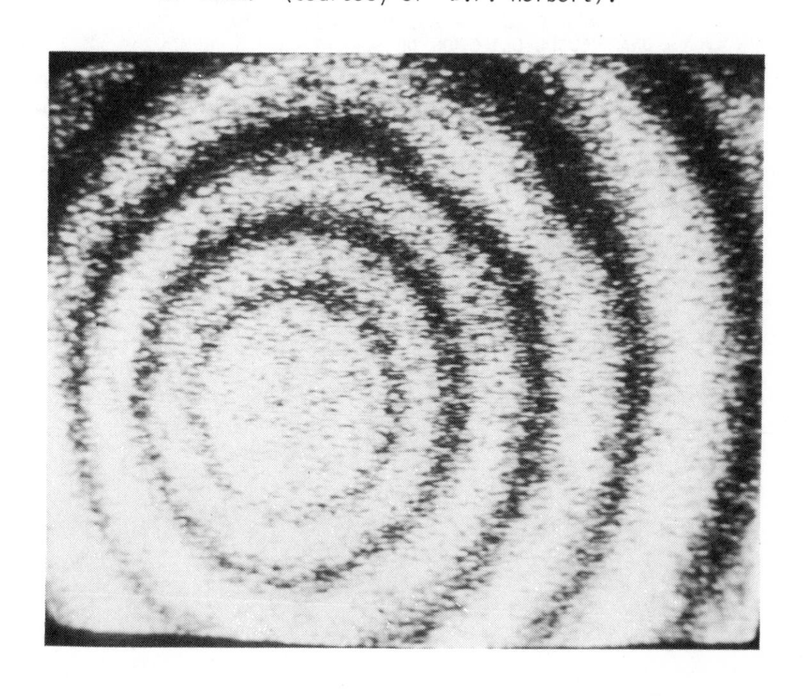

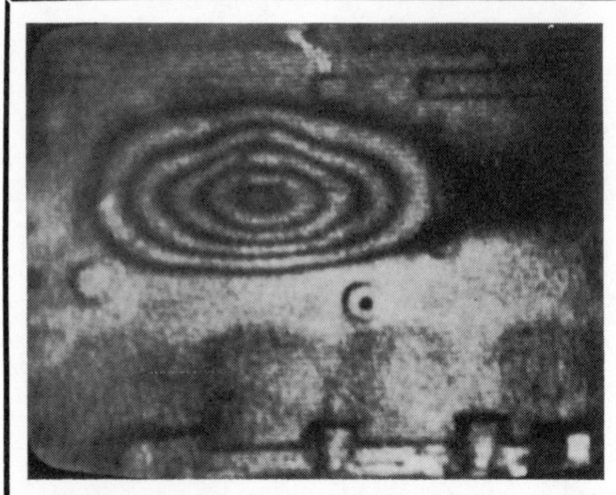

SINGLE RESONANT SITE ON ENGINE SIDE WALL AFTER ENHANCEMENT AND STROBING WITHOUT PHASE DETAIL

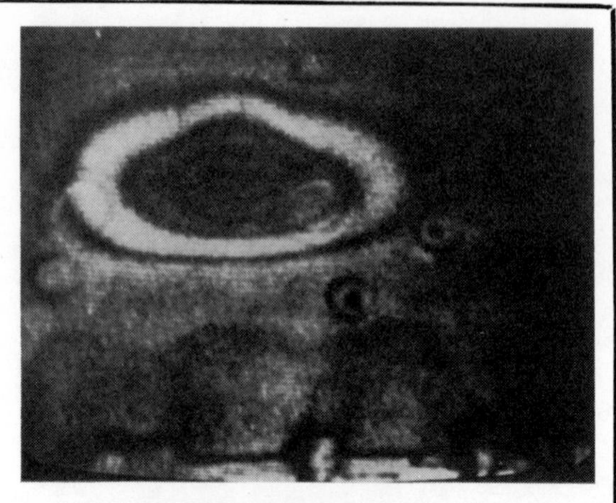

SINGLE RESONANT SITE
WITH OPTICAL PHASE DELAY INTRODUCED
TO SHOW RELATIVE PHASE OF VIBRATION MODE

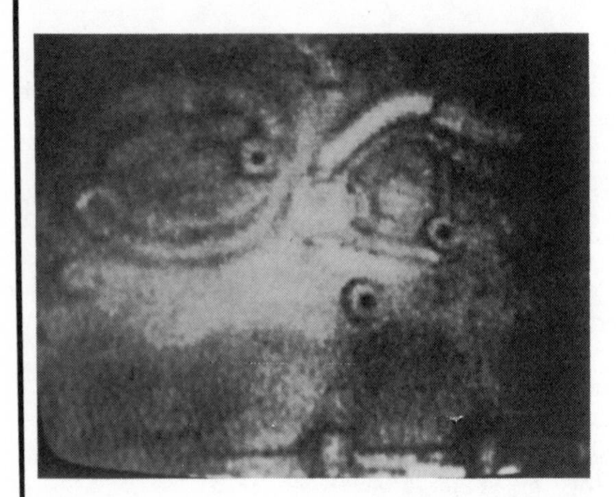

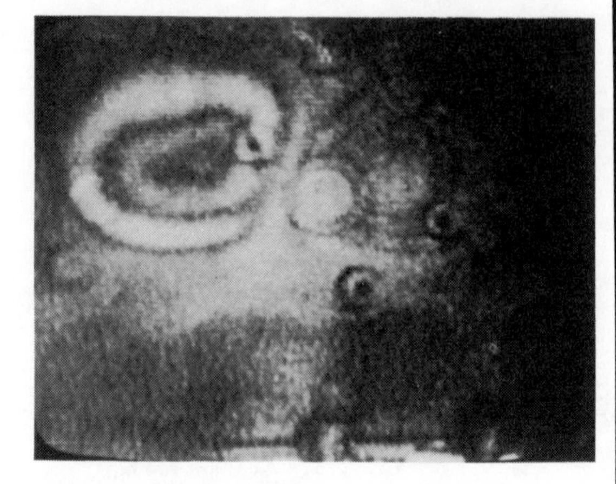

DOUBLE RESONANT VIBRATION SITE ON SIDE WALL OF ENGINE
WITH OPTICAL PHASE DELAY TO ALLOW
UNAMBIGUOUS DETECTION OF SURFACE DISPLACEMENT

Fig. 3.7. Engine results with phase delay.

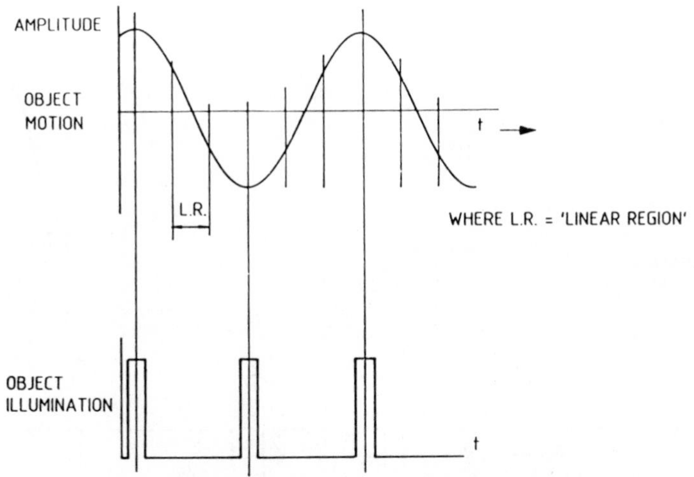

CASE 1. STROBOSCOPE ILLUMINATION FOR MAXIMUM DIPLACEMENT

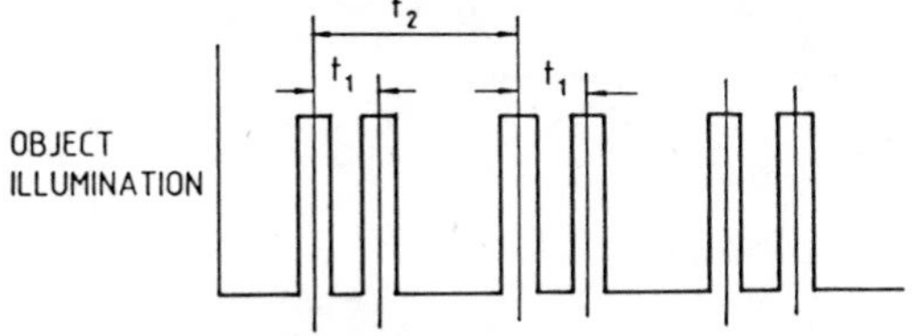

CASE 2. STROBOSCOPE ILLUMINATION FOR SAMPLED DISPLACEMENT

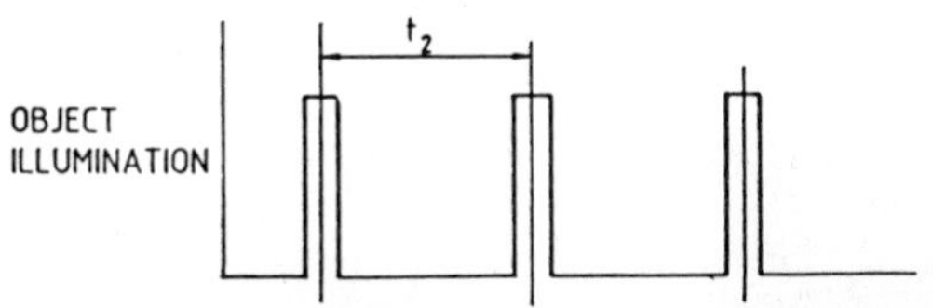

CASE 3. STROBOSCOPE ILLUMINATION TO ACHIEVE SAME CONDITIONS AS CASE 2

FIG. 3.8 STROBOSCOPE ILLUMINATION

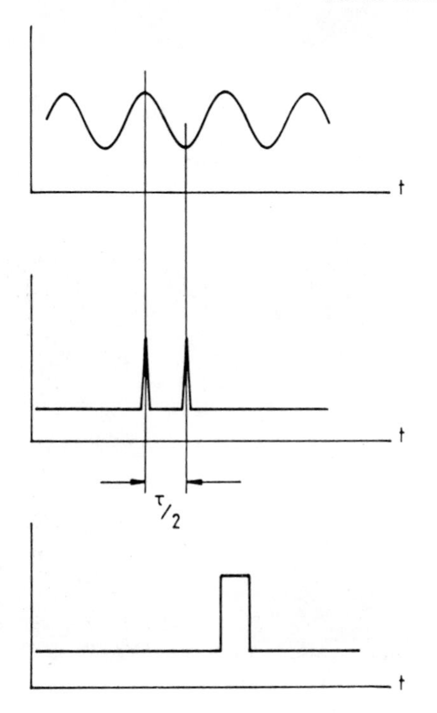

STRUCTURE RESPONCE

LASER FIRING, TRIGGERED TO COINSIDE WITH THE PEAKS OF DISPLACEMENT,(THIS CAN BE MODIFIED)

THE T.V. CAMERA IS BLANKED PRIOR TO LASER FIRING AND IS ADDRESSED AFTER THE TWO LASER PULSES WHEN ONLY COMBINED IMAGE IS READ FROM THE IMAGING TUBE AND STORED DIGITALLY

FIG.3.9 DOUBLE PULSED E.S.P.I. OPERATION

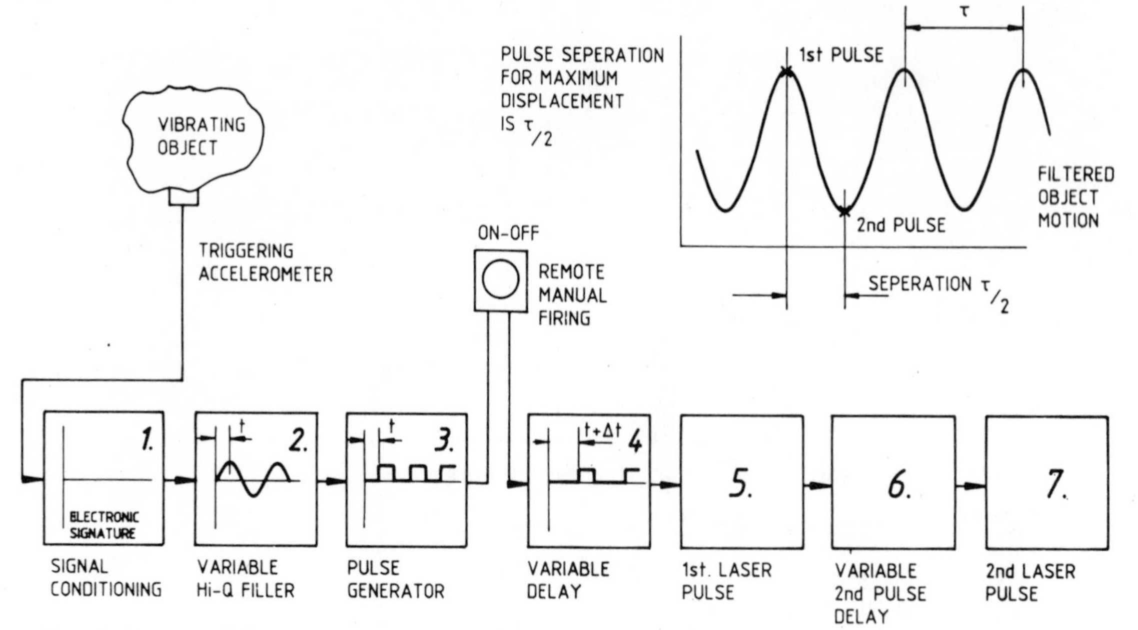

Fig. 3.10. Laser control and firing system.

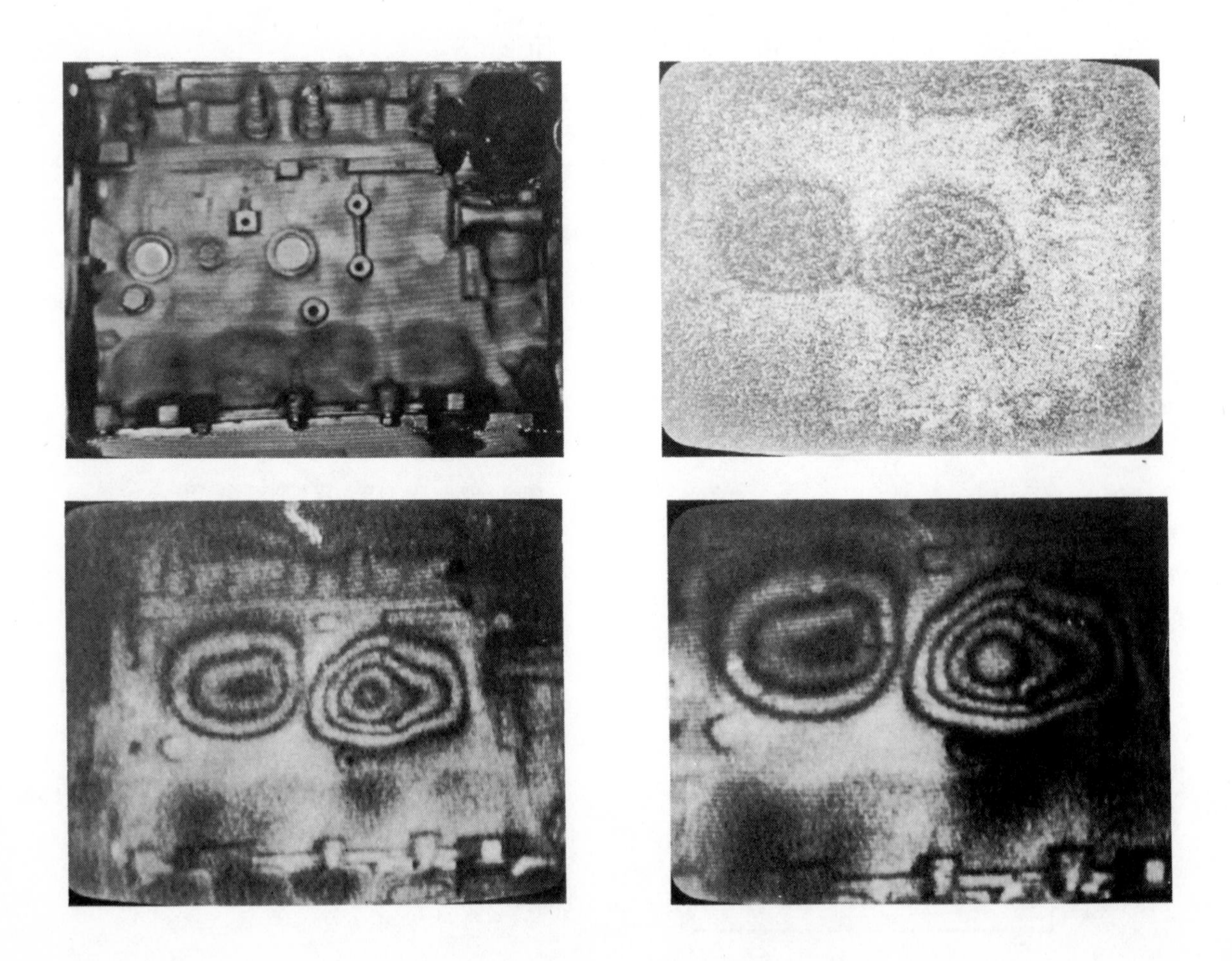

Fig. 4.1. Use of speckle averaging and zoom imaging lenses for enhanced fringe visibility and interogation.

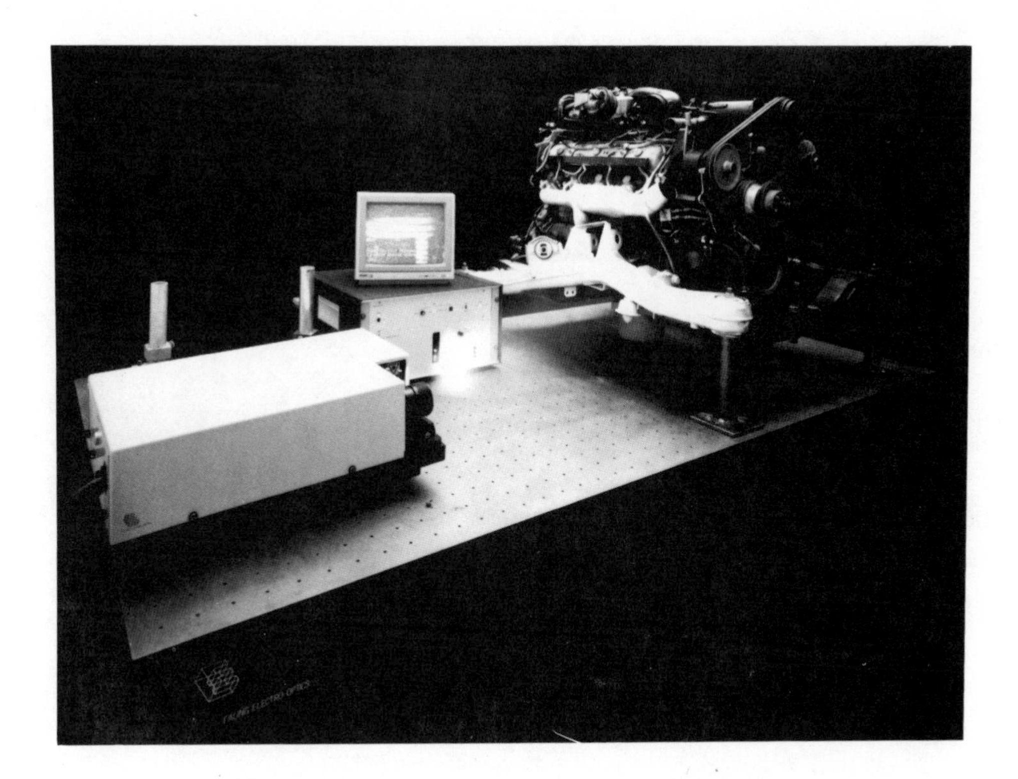

Fig. 4.2 The Vidispec system manufactured by Ealing Electro-Optics working on a large motor car engine and sub-frame at the Deptartment of Mechanical Engineering, Loughborough University of Technology.

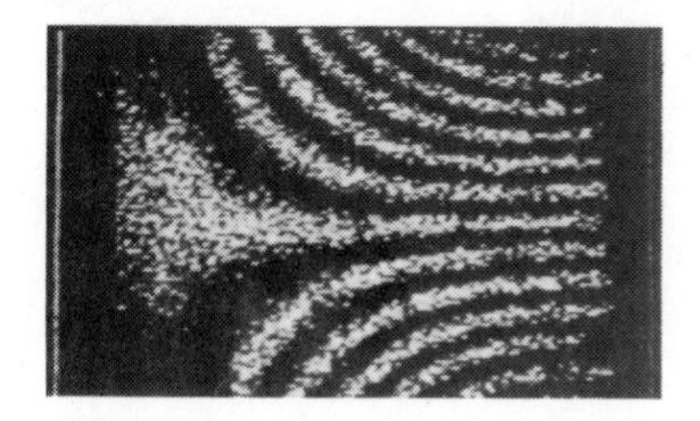
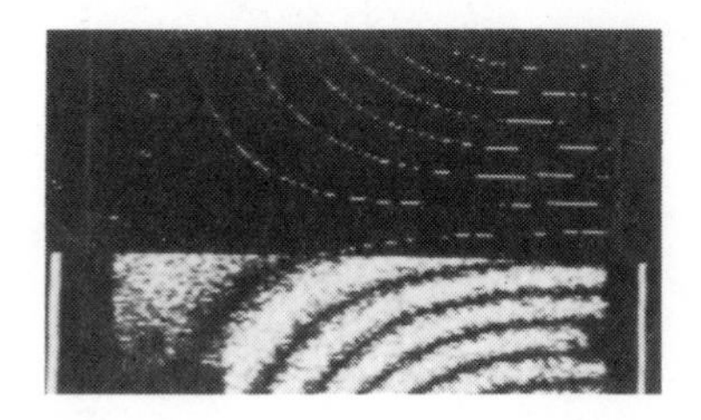
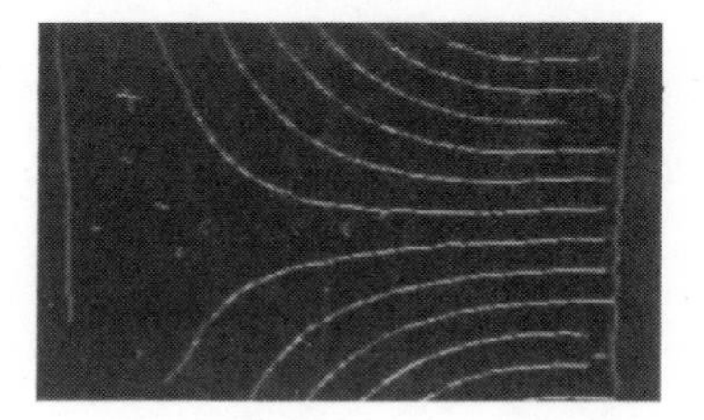

Fig. 4.3. Automatic fringe tracking. (Courtesy of P Henry)

HOLOGRAPHIC NONDESTRUCTIVE TESTING:
STATUS AND COMPARISON WITH CONVENTIONAL METHODS

Volume 604

Addendum

The following papers were presented at this conference, but the manuscripts supporting the oral presentations are not available.

[604-02] **Product needs for practical holography**
A. Gara, Newport Corp.

[604-05] **Holographic NDT of rotating machinery**
W. F. Fagan, Jurid Werke GmbH, West Germany

AUTHOR INDEX